Workbook for
Successful Nursing Assistant Care

SECOND EDITION

Hartman Publishing, Inc. **hartman**online.com

CREDITS

Managing Editor
Susan Alvare

Developmental Editor
Suzanne Wegner

Cover Designer
Kirsten Browne

Interior Designer
Thaddeus Castillo

Composition
Thaddeus Castillo

Proofreaders
Kristin Calderon
Leslie McMurtry

NOTICE TO READERS

Though the guidelines and procedures contained in this text are based on consultations with healthcare professionals, they should not be considered absolute recommendations. The instructor and readers should follow employer, local, state, and federal guidelines concerning healthcare practices. These guidelines change, and it is the reader's responsibility to be aware of these changes and of the policies and procedures of her or his healthcare facility.

The publisher, author, editors, and reviewers cannot accept any responsibility for errors or omissions or for any consequences from application of the information in this book and make no warranty, expressed or implied, with respect to the contents of the book. The Publisher does not warrant or guarantee any of the products described herein or perform any analysis in connection with any of the product information contained herein.

COPYRIGHT INFORMATION

ISBN 10 1-888343-98-2

ISBN 13 978-1-888343-98-4

preface

Welcome to the Workbook!

This workbook is designed to help you review what you have learned from reading your textbook. For this reason, the workbook is organized around learning objectives, just like your textbook and even your instructor's teaching material. Including the learning objectives makes it easier for you to go back and reread a section if you need to refresh your memory.

These learning objectives work as a built-in study guide. After completing the exercises for each learning objective in the workbook, ask yourself if you can DO what that learning objective describes.

If you can, move on to the next learning objective. If you cannot, just go back to the textbook, reread that learning objective, and try again.

We have provided procedure checklists, as well as a practice exam for the certification test, at the end of the workbook. The answers to the workbook exercises are in your instructor's teaching guide.

Happy Learning!

Table of Contents

1
The Nursing Assistant in Long-Term Care

1. Review the key terms in Learning Objective 1 before completing the workbook exercises

2. Describe healthcare settings

Multiple Choice.
Circle the letter of the correct answer.

1. Another name for a long-term care (LTC) facility is:
   a. Nursing home
   b. Home health care
   c. Assisted living facility
   d. Adult daycare facility

2. People who live in long-term care facilities are called residents because:
   a. The facility is their home.
   b. They are picked up at the end of each day to go home.
   c. They do not have any living family members.
   d. They do not need skilled care.

3. Assisted living facilities are initially for:
   a. Residents who need around-the-clock intensive care
   b. Residents who are generally independent and do not need skilled care
   c. Residents who will die within six months
   d. Residents who need to be in an acute care facility

4. Home health care differs from nursing assistant care in this way:
   a. Home health aides do not have to assist with personal care.
   b. Home health aides may clean the home and do laundry.
   c. Home health aides do not have supervisors.
   d. Home health care takes place in a hospital, rather than a long-term care facility.

5. Care given by a specialist to restore or improve function after an illness or injury is called:
   a. Acute care
   b. Subacute care
   c. Rehabilitation
   d. Hospice care

6. Inter-generational care is:
   a. People of the same generation spending time together
   b. Pets brought into the facility to help brighten a resident's day
   c. Adult and child daycare merged so that young and old can spend time together
   d. The generation caring for children and aging parents at the same time

3. Explain Medicare and Medicaid

True or False.
Circle the "T" for true or the "F" for false for each of the following statements.

1. T F Medicare is a health insurance program for people who are 65 years of age or older.

2. T F No one younger than 65 is covered by Medicare.

3. T F Medicare will pay for any services requested by the resident.

4. T F A person with limited income might qualify for Medicaid.

5. T F Medicare and Medicaid pay a fixed amount for services based on residents' needs.

4. Describe the residents for whom you will care

True or False.

1. T F It is more important to know residents individually than to know general facts about most residents.

2. T F Most residents are male.

3. T F Residents with the longest average stay in a healthcare facility are residents admitted for rehabilitation or terminal care.

4. T F Dementia is not a major cause of admission to a nursing home.

5. T F Disorders themselves are not the only reason residents are admitted to long-term care facilities. Often they are admitted due to lack of a support system.

6. T F Lack of outside support for many residents is one reason to care for the "whole person" instead of only the illness or disease.

5. Describe the nursing assistant's role

Short Answer.
Answer each of the following questions in the space provided.

1. Define delegation.

_____

_____

_____

_____

2. Think of one task that might be delegated to a nursing assistant that is not mentioned in the book.

_____

_____

_____

_____

_____

3. List seven tasks performed by nursing assistants. Which task do you think you will enjoy the most? Which do you think will be the hardest for you?

_____

_____

_____

_____

_____

_____

_____

_____

_____

_____

6. Discuss professionalism and list examples of professional behavior

Multiple Choice.

1. All of the following are true of professionalism EXCEPT:
   a. Nursing assistants should address residents in the way they wish to be addressed.
   b. Nursing assistants should discuss personal problems with residents.
   c. Dressing appropriately is part of professionalism.
   d. Professional behavior includes being on time for work and avoiding unnecessary absences.

2. Katie is a new nursing assistant at Parkwood facility and wants to make a good first impression. What is one thing she can do to show professionalism at her new job?
   a. Ignore any constructive criticism she receives from others.
   b. Tell a resident about another resident's condition.
   c. Ask questions when she does not understand something.
   d. Address the residents by using affectionate nicknames like "Honey" or "Granny."

7. List qualities that nursing assistants must have

Scenarios.
Read each of the following scenarios and answer the questions that follow.

Nursing assistant Samantha Stevens is late for five shifts in a row. On the fifth day, her supervisor asks her about this. Samantha replies, "It's not my fault. Traffic has been horrible, and I just wish this facility was on a more convenient street."

1. How could Samantha have been more humble and open to growth?

_____

_____

_____

_____

_____

_____

Nurse Frederico Gonzalez tells nursing assistant Mary Lupko about a resident's diagnosis of a sexually-transmitted disease. He gives specific instructions about the resident's care. Mary sees a fellow nursing assistant across the hall, and says, "How do you think Joann Timbly got an STD? Her husband hasn't visited in months."

2. How could Mary have been more trustworthy?

_____

_____

_____

_____

_____

_____

Nursing assistant Rob Brown is tidying Ms. Lee's room. He notices a Buddha statue and asks, "Why don't you believe in Christ? Christianity is the only real religion."

3. How could Rob have acted in a courteous and respectful manner?

_____

_____

_____

_____

_____

_____

Resident Hannah Stein is dying. She tells nursing assistant Jennifer Wells that she always wanted to be nicer to her son and to have a better relationship. Jennifer replies, "Yeah, well, you think you got it hard? My son won't even talk to me because I wouldn't let him go to a basketball game on a school night." Then Jennifer proceeds to tell Mrs. Stein about her divorce and how her son's father never helps out.

4. How could Jennifer have been more empathetic?

_____

_____

_____

_____

_____

_____

_____

_____

_____

Nursing assistant Doug Albin is helping resident Sam Perkins to the bathroom. Sam walks slowly and has to rely on his walker for help. Doug notices that his shift is over in five minutes. Doug says, "Can't you walk a little faster? I'm outta here in five minutes!"

5. How could Doug have been more patient and understanding?

_____

_____

_____

_____

_____

_____

_____

_____

_____

_____

Nursing assistant Wayne Leach just found out his facility is short-staffed tonight, and he will have to help five additional residents get ready for bed. "Oh great," he says. "Now I'll never get this done!"

6. How could Wayne have been more enthusiastic?

_____

_____

_____

_____

_____

_____

_____

_____

Nurse Cathy Connell verbally gives nursing assistant Sandra Levy a list of things she wants done. Sandra simply says, "Okay" and walks off. As she turns the corner, she forgets what Nurse Connell wanted her to do first. "Oh well," she shrugs. "I'm sure it's not the end of the world."

7. How could Sandra have been more dependable?

_____

_____

_____

_____

_____

_____

_____

Nursing assistant Tracy Fleming is assigned to help Mr. Ming, a resident from China, eat his dinner. Even though she has never met Mr. Ming, she complains, "I hate helping Asian residents! I can never understand anything they are saying."

8. How could Tracy have shown more tolerance and lack of prejudice?

_____

_____

_____

_____

_____

_____

_____

_____

_____

8. Discuss proper grooming guidelines

True or False.

1. T F Long hair should be kept down around the face while giving care to residents.

2. T F False nails harbor bacteria no matter how well hands are washed.

3. T F Wearing strong scents or perfumes at work is a good idea.

4. T F Big hoop earrings can be worn around residents who will not pull them out.

5. T F A nursing assistant should wear light makeup or none at all.

6. T F Long nails are fine to have, as long as they're not false nails.

7. T F Jewelry can collect bacteria.

8. T F A nursing assistant only needs to bathe or shower three times a week.

9. Define the roles of each member of the care team

Matching.
Write the letter of the correct description beside each care team member listed below.

a. Person who determines residents' needs and helps them get support services, such as counseling and financial assistance

b. Person who is the most important part of the care team

c. Person who gives therapy in the form of heat, cold, massage, ultrasound, electricity and exercise to improve circulation, promote healing, ease pain, and improve mobility

d. Person who performs many assigned tasks, such as bathing residents, and assisting with toileting; the person who usually has the most direct contact with residents

e. Person who teaches exercises to help residents improve or overcome speech problems; also evaluates ability to swallow food and drink

f. Person who assesses resident status, monitors progress, and gives treatments; may be NA's supervisor

g. Person who diagnoses disease or disability and prescribes treatment

h. Person who assesses the resident's nutritional status and plans a program of nutritional care

i. Person who works with people who need help with activities of daily living

j. Person who plans activities for residents to help them socialize and stay active

1. _____ Registered dietician

2. _____ Physician

3. _____ Occupational therapist

4. _____ Medical social worker

5. _____ Activities director

6. _____ Speech language pathologist

7. _____ Nurse

8. _____ Resident

9. _____ Nursing assistant

10. _____ Physical therapist

10. Discuss the facility chain of command

Fill in the Blank.
Fill in the correct word in each blank below.

1. The chain of command describes the line of

_____

in a facility.

2. The _____ will usually be the nursing assistant's immediate supervisor.

3. When a nursing assistant has a problem with another department, it should be reported to an immediate supervisor or the _____ nurse.

4. Following the chain of command protects staff from _____, which is a legal term for being held responsible for harming someone else.

11. Explain "The Five Rights of Delegation"

Short Answer.

1. What are three questions nurses consider before delegating a task?

_____

_____

_____

_____

_____

_____

_____

_____

_____

_____

_____

_____

2. What are three questions nursing assistants should ask themselves before accepting a delegation?

_____

_____

_____

_____

_____

_____

3. If a nursing assistant is unsure about a task that is delegated to him, what should he do?

_____

_____

_____

_____

12. Describe four methods of nursing care

Matching.

a. Method of care in which the resident is the primary focus and is able to see many of the same people perform the care

b. Method of care in which a nurse acts as the team leader of a group of individuals giving care

c. Method of care assigning specific tasks to each team member

d. Method of care in which the registered nurse gives much of the daily care to residents

1. ____ Team nursing

2. ____ Functional nursing

3. ____ Resident-focused care

4. ____ Primary nursing

13. Explain policy and procedure manuals

Fill in the Blank.

1. A _____ is a course of action that to be taken every time a certain situation occurs.

2. A complete list of every facility policy is found in the _____.

3. A _____ is a specific way of doing something.

4. The exact way to complete every resident procedure is found in the _____.

5. Nursing assistants who _____ _____ when they are unsure provide safer care.

14. Describe the long-term care survey process

True or False.

1. T F A survey is conducted by a team of professionals to make sure long-term care facilities are following state and federal regulations.

2. T F If a surveyor asks a nursing assistant a question and she does not know the answer, she should quickly make one up.

3. T F Surveyors will interview residents to get their opinions about the care they receive.

4. T F Membership in The Joint Commission is mandatory for all healthcare facilities.

2
Ethical and Legal Issues

1. Review the key terms in Learning Objective 1 before completing the workbook exercises

2. Define the terms "law," "ethics," and "etiquette"

Multiple Choice.
Circle the letter of the correct answer.

1. The knowledge of right and wrong are:
    a. Ethics
    b. Civil laws
    c. Etiquette
    d. Criminal laws

2. Which of the following is a law?
    a. A nursing assistant must not gossip about residents or other staff members.
    b. A nursing assistant must be polite when answering the telephone.
    c. A nursing assistant must not steal residents' belongings.
    d. A nursing assistant must not discuss personal problems with co-workers.

3. Laws to protect society from people or organizations that try to do them harm are:
    a. Civil laws
    b. Criminal laws
    c. Felonies
    d. Misdemeanors

4. A code of courtesy and proper behavior in a certain setting is called:
    a. Civil law
    b. Criminal law
    c. Ethics
    d. Etiquette

3. Discuss examples of ethical and professional behavior

Crossword Puzzle.
Fill in each of the blanks below and use your answers to complete the crossword puzzle.

Across.

2. If a nursing assistant makes a mistake, it is important to _____ it immediately.

4. A _____ person is empathetic with a person who is ill and respects the ill person's beliefs.

5. _____ care given accurately and promptly.

7. Report _____ of residents.

8. A nursing assistant must keep all resident information

    _____.

Down.

1. A person who is cheerful and

    _____ is someone others like to be around.

3. _____ others is important in facilities.

6. The ability to understand what is proper and appropriate when dealing with others is called _____.

9. _____ means sharing in the feelings and troubles of others.

4. Describe a nursing assistant code of ethics

Short Answer.

Answer each of the following questions in the space provided.

1. What is one way that a nursing assistant can make sure she keeps up with new information on the job?

_____

_____

_____

_____

_____

2. What are two ways you plan to show a positive attitude toward residents, staff and visitors when you start your new job?

_____

_____

_____

_____

_____

_____

_____

3. What is one way to help preserve resident safety?

_____

_____

_____

_____

_____

_____

_____

_____

4. If a nursing assistant suspects that a resident is being abused, what should she do?

_____

_____

_____

_____

_____

_____

5. Explain the Omnibus Budget Reconciliation Act (OBRA)

Multiple Choice.

1. Why was the Omnibus Budget Reconciliation Act (OBRA) passed in 1987?
   a. As a response to reports of poor care and abuse in nursing homes
   b. Because of complaints by nursing assistants of uncooperative residents
   c. To control costs in nursing homes
   d. Because most nursing homes employed too many nursing assistants

2. How does the OBRA law relate to nursing assistants?
   a. Tests nursing assistants' knowledge of care procedures
   b. Sets minimum requirements for training, competency exams, and in-service education
   c. Outlines specific steps for handling infectious material
   d. The OBRA law does not apply to nursing assistants

3. How many hours of training must nursing assistants complete before working to meet OBRA requirements?
   a. 30 hours
   b. 50 hours
   c. 75 hours
   d. 100 hours

4. All of the following are a part of OBRA's regulations EXCEPT:
   a. Identify rights for residents in nursing homes
   b. Standardized training of nursing assistants
   c. Complete assessments of every resident
   d. Steps to follow if a nursing assistant is exposed to a bloodborne pathogen

6. Explain Residents' Rights

Short Answer.
For each of the following Residents' Rights, give one example of how a nursing assistant can respect that right on the job.

1. The right to the best quality of life possible

   _____

   _____

   _____

   _____

   _____

2. The right to receive the correct care in the form of services and activities to maintain a high level of wellness

   _____

   _____

   _____

   _____

   _____

3. The right to be fully informed about rights and services

   _____

   _____

   _____

   _____

   _____

   _____

4. The right to participate in their own care

   _____

   _____

   _____

   _____

   _____

5. The right to make independent choices

   _____

   _____

   _____

   _____

   _____

6. The right to privacy and confidentiality

   _____

   _____

   _____

   _____

   _____

7. The right to dignity, respect, and freedom

   _____

   _____

   _____

Name: _____

8. The right to security of possessions

_____

_____

_____

_____

_____

9. Rights with transfers and discharges

_____

_____

_____

_____

_____

10. The right to complain

_____

_____

_____

_____

_____

11. The right to visits

_____

_____

_____

_____

_____

7. Explain types of abuse and neglect

Matching.
Write the letter of the correct definition beside each term.

a. Actions or failure to act or give care resulting in injury to a person

b. The use of legal or illegal drugs, cigarettes or alcohol in a way that harms oneself or others

c. Any unwelcome sexual advance or behavior that creates an intimidating or hostile work environment

d. Intentionally harming a person physically, mentally, or emotionally by failing to give needed or correct care

e. Confinement or separation from others without consent

f. Unlawfully restraining or confining someone, or threatening to do so

g. Physical or verbal abuse of staff by other staff, residents or visitors

h. Touching a person without his or her permission

i. Threatening to touch a person without his or her permission

j. Stealing or improperly using the money or other assets of another

k. Forcing a person to perform or participate in sexual acts

l. Oral or written words, pictures or gestures that threaten or embarrass another person

m. Harming a person by threatening, scaring, insulting or humiliating him or her

n. Abuse by spouses, intimate partners, or family members

o. Purposely causing physical, mental, or emotional pain or injury to someone

p. Intentional or unintentional treatment that causes harm to a person's body

q. Unintentionally harming a person physically, mentally, or emotionally by failing to give needed or correct care

Name: _____

1. _____ Abuse

2. _____ Active neglect

3. _____ Assault

4. _____ Battery

5. _____ Domestic violence

6. _____ False imprisonment

7. _____ Financial abuse

8. _____ Involuntary seclusion

9. _____ Negligence

10. _____ Passive neglect

11. _____ Physical abuse

12. _____ Psychological abuse

13. _____ Sexual abuse

14. _____ Sexual harassment

15. _____ Substance abuse

16. _____ Verbal abuse

17. _____ Workplace violence

Multiple Choice.

1. What should a nursing assistant do if he sees or suspects that a resident is being abused?
   a. Report it to the supervisor and document it at once.
   b. Keep watching the resident to make sure he is correct.
   c. Ignore it until the resident complains about it.
   d. Confront the abuser.

2. If a resident wants to make a complaint of abuse, the nursing assistant's responsibility is to:
   a. Confirm that abuse has really occurred before reporting it.
   b. Assist the resident in every possible way.
   c. Retaliate against the resident for making a complaint.
   d. Ask other residents if they have seen any abuse occurring.

3. An example of sexual abuse is:
   a. A nursing assistant does not respond to a call light.
   b. A nursing assistant shows a resident a pornographic magazine.
   c. A nursing assistant leaves a resident alone in his room and does not check on him.
   d. A nursing assistant screams at a resident.

4. An example of financial abuse is:
   a. A nursing assistant loudly announces in the hallway that a resident has "wet his bed again."
   b. A nursing assistant makes fun of a resident's religion.
   c. A nursing assistant sells crafts that a resident has made for profit and keeps the money.
   d. A nursing assistant hits a resident.

5. An example of psychological abuse is:
   a. A nursing assistant roughly hurries a resident to the bathroom.
   b. A nursing assistant tells a resident he needs money for school.
   c. A nursing assistant forces a resident to rub up against her.
   d. While giving care to a resident, a nursing assistant tells him he smells bad.

8. Recognize signs and symptoms of abuse and neglect

True or False.
Circle the "T" for true or the "F" for false for each of the following statements.

1. T F Ignoring a call light is not considered abuse or neglect.

2. T F Unexplained broken bones, burns, and bruising are all signs of abuse.

3. T F Lack of appetite and weight loss can be signs of abuse.

4. T F Similar injuries that occur over and over probably just mean that the resident is clumsy.

5. T F If a resident shows fear or anxiety when a certain caregiver is present, this may be a sign of abuse.

6. T F Mood swings and depression are always caused by illness or chemical imbalance.

7. T F If a resident is unclean or has a strong smell of urine, it probably just means he does not like to bathe.

8. T F Sores on the body can indicate neglect.

9. T F If a resident's family is concerned that abuse is occurring, it is considered a possible sign of abuse.

10. T F If a nursing assistant only suspects abuse, she should wait until she is sure it is happening before reporting it.

9. Describe the steps taken if a nursing assistant is suspected of abuse

Multiple Choice.

1. What is the first thing that happens when a report of nursing assistant abuse has been made?
   a. The NA is immediately fired.
   b. The NA is immediately suspended.
   c. The NA is allowed to keep working until the investigation is completed.
   d. The NA is transferred to another facility.

2. Which of the following is NOT one of the steps followed by the Nurse Aide Training and Competency Evaluation Program (NATCEP) when a claim of abuse is made?
   a. Investigation
   b. Notification
   c. Relocation of the resident
   d. A hearing

3. If the claim of abuse is proven to be true, what happens?
   a. The NA is placed in the abuse registry in addition to other possible penalties.
   b. The resident is moved to another facility.
   c. The NA is transferred to another facility.
   d. The facility is cited for negligence.

10. Discuss the ombudsman's role

Short Answer.

1. What is the role of an ombudsman?

_____

_____

_____

_____

_____

_____

_____

_____

_____

_____

_____

2. Which other people or organizations can a resident or his family contact for help or to make a complaint?

_____

_____

_____

_____

_____

_____

11. Explain HIPAA and related terms

Multiple Choice.

1. Why was the Health Insurance Portability and Accountability Act (HIPAA) created?
   a. To protect the privacy of health information
   b. To reduce instances of abuse in facilities
   c. To address infection control issues
   d. To ensure adequate training for nursing assistants

2. Who may have access to private health information (PHI) about a resident?
   a. Anyone who asks
   b. Only the resident's friends and family
   c. Only people who must have the information for care or to process records
   d. No one

3. If a person who is not directly involved in a resident's care asks a nursing assistant for PHI, how should the nursing assistant respond?
   a. Ignore them.
   b. Ask the supervisor what to tell them.
   c. Say, "I cannot share that information. It is confidential."
   d. Tell them, but ask them not to tell anyone about it.

4. All of the following are ways to keep health information confidential EXCEPT:
   a. Do not discuss residents in public areas.
   b. Do not include private information in e-mails.
   c. Double-check fax numbers and always use a cover sheet.
   d. Bring family to the facility to meet the residents.

5. All of the following are considered invasion of privacy EXCEPT:
   a. A nursing assistant telling her husband about a resident's recent diagnosis of cancer
   b. A nursing assistant telling her supervisor that a resident may be developing pressure sores
   c. Showing a picture of a resident to a neighbor
   d. Telling a local newspaper about a celebrity who had been admitted to nursing home

12. Discuss the Patient Self-Determination Act (PSDA) and advance directives

True or False.

1. T F A DNR order tells healthcare professionals to keep trying to resuscitate a resident if his heart stops.

2. T F The Patient Self-Determination Act encourages people to make decisions about advance directives.

3. T F Advance directives designate the kind of care people want in the event they are unable to make those decisions themselves.

4. T F A Living Will designates the people who will inherit the resident's estate if he or she dies.

5. T F A Durable Power of Attorney for Health Care appoints a person to make medical decisions for a resident if he or she becomes unable to do so.

6. T F A person is legally required to have advance directives.

7. T F Facilities are required by Medicare and Medicaid to give residents and staff information about rights relating to advance directives.

3
Communication Skills

1. Review the key terms in Learning Objective 1 before completing the workbook exercises

2. Explain types of communication

True or False.
Circle the "T" for true or the "F" for false for each of the following statements.

1. T F People communicate with words, drawings, pictures and behavior.

2. T F The receiver and sender never switch roles during communication.

3. T F Speaking and writing are two examples of verbal communication.

4. T F How a person's voice sounds and the words he chooses are not important during communication.

5. T F Nonverbal communication includes posture and facial expressions.

6. T F Making positive changes in body language will improve communication.

7. T F It is a good idea for a nursing assistant to finish a resident's sentences for him to show that she understands what he is telling her.

8. T F Use mostly facts when communicating.

Fill in the Blank.
For each of the following behaviors, decide whether it's an example of positive or negative nonverbal communication. Write "P" for positive or "N" for negative.

1. ____ Smiling and nodding

2. ____ Crossing arms

3. ____ Looking away while someone is talking

4. ____ Leaning forward to listen

5. ____ Pointing at someone while speaking

6. ____ Rolling eyes

7. ____ With permission, putting a hand over a resident's hand while listening to her

8. ____ Tapping a foot

3. Explain barriers to communication

Scenarios.
Read the following scenarios and answer the questions.

Nursing assistant Barbara Smith thinks resident Mrs. Gold is in pain. Barbara asks her if she is okay. Before Mrs. Gold answers, Barbara looks around the room and begins to gather her supplies to leave. Mrs. Gold simply says, "Yes."

1. Identify the barrier to communication occurring here and suggest a way to avoid it.

_____

_____

_____

_____

_____

_____

_____

Resident Marla Gibson had a stroke that affects her speech. She asks her nursing assistant for a glass of water. The nursing assistant replies, "I have no idea where your daughter is," and leaves the room.

16

Name: _____

2. Identify the barrier to communication occurring here and suggest a way to avoid it.

_____

_____

_____

_____

_____

_____

_____

_____

_____

_____

_____

_____

_____

Nursing assistant Kena Wright asks resident Josiah Crane, "You have NKA, right?" He nods. She reports to the nurse, who looks over his chart. "No, that's not true," the nurse says. "He is allergic to penicillin. I wonder why he told you that."

3. Identify the barrier to communication occurring here and suggest a way to avoid it.

_____

_____

_____

_____

_____

_____

_____

_____

Nursing assistant Jerry Wells sees that resident Eli Levine is having difficulty moving his leg after his total hip replacement surgery. Jerry says, "You should start doing range of motion exercises right away and bearing as much weight as possible." Mr. Levine attempts to stand on his leg and screams in pain.

4. Identify the barrier to communication occurring here and suggest a way to avoid it.

Resident Paul Jackson is at risk for dehydration. Nursing assistants are asked to encourage him to drink as much as possible. To find out what Mr. Jackson likes to drink, nursing assistant Gracie Truman asks him, "Do you like orange juice?" He says, "No."

5. Identify the barrier to communication occurring here and suggest a way to avoid it.

_____

_____

_____

_____

_____

_____

_____

Nursing assistant Lyla Cooper is helping resident Josie Bayer get ready to attend a guest lecture with another resident. Josie says, "I don't want to go with her." Lyla asks, "Why?" Josie replies, "I just don't."

6. Identify the barrier to communication occurring here and suggest a way to avoid it.

_____

_____

Name: _____

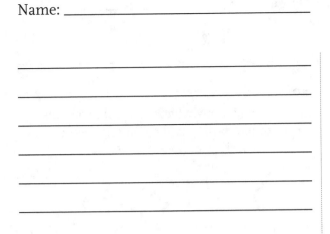

Nursing assistant Tracy Fleming is assigned to give Mr. Perez, who speaks very little English, a bed bath. She explains the procedure, and Mr. Perez nods even though he looks a little confused. When she starts to take off his shirt, he gets very upset.

7. Identify the barrier to communication occurring here and suggest a way to avoid it.

_____

_____

_____

_____

_____

_____

_____

_____

4. List ways that cultures impact communication

Multiple Choice.
Circle the letter of the correct answer.

1. Which of the following is NOT true of culture?
   a. A culture is a set of learned beliefs, values and behaviors.
   b. The use of touch and eye contact varies in different cultures.
   c. There are only a few cultures in the world.
   d. Cultures communicate in many different ways.

2. If a resident seems to be sensitive to eye contact and/or touch, a nursing assistant should:
   a. Make eye contact and touch him as much as possible so that he gets used to it.
   b. Respect his wishes and limit eye contact and touch as much as possible.
   c. Explain to the resident that we do things differently in our culture and he needs to adapt.
   d. Ignore the sensitivity and use eye contact and touch as with any other resident.

3. Which of the following is UNACCEPTABLE touch when working with residents?
   a. Sitting on a resident's lap if asked to
   b. Giving respectful personal care
   c. Hugging with permission
   d. Holding a resident's hand if asked

4. One good way for a nursing assistant to deal with a language barrier with a resident is to:
   a. Use an interpreter
   b. Teach the resident words in the nursing assistant's language
   c. Speak with other staff in the nursing assistant's language in front of the resident
   d. Get someone else to care for the resident

5. Identify the people you will communicate with in a facility

True or False.

1. T F When a nursing assistant first greets a resident, he should introduce himself and identify the resident.

2. T F In the facility, a nursing assistant may communicate by charting, using a computer, or on the telephone.

3. T F If a nursing assistant has performed a procedure for a resident before, she doesn't need to explain it the next time she does it.

4. T F Communication with other departments within a facility is not common and is unimportant.

Name: _____

5. T F One way to let a resident's family know that staff are providing excellent care for him or her is to always answer call lights promptly.

6. T F Families can provide valuable information about a resident's preferences and histories.

7. T F If a doctor's office calls and asks for information about a resident, the nursing assistant should give it to them.

6. Understand basic medical terminology and abbreviations

Matching.
Write the letter of the correct definition beside each term listed below.

a. The main part of a word

b. A word part placed at the end of a word

c. A word part added to the beginning of a word

d. A shortened word

1. _____ Abbreviation

2. _____ Root

3. _____ Suffix

4. _____ Prefix

Short Answer.
Answer the following questions in the space provided.

1. When is it appropriate to use medical terminology on the job? When is it inappropriate?

_____
_____
_____
_____
_____
_____
_____
_____
_____

_____
_____

2. How will knowledge of the abbreviations used in a facility make a nursing assistant's job easier?

_____
_____
_____
_____
_____
_____
_____
_____
_____
_____
_____

7. Explain how to convert regular time to military time

Fill in the Blank.
Fill in the correct time in each of the blanks.

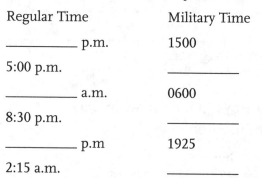

Regular Time	Military Time
_____ p.m.	1500
5:00 p.m.	_____
_____ a.m.	0600
8:30 p.m.	_____
_____ p.m	1925
2:15 a.m.	_____

8. Describe a standard resident chart

Multiple Choice.

1. The nursing assistant's responsibility when charting in a medical record includes:
   a. Making changes in residents' diets
   b. Changing medications
   c. Gathering information and reporting to the nurse
   d. Creating a new exercise plan

Name: _____

2. Which of the following information would NOT be found on a resident's chart?
   a. Advance directives
   b. Intake and output records
   c. Care plans
   d. Information about the resident's room-mate

9. Explain guidelines for documentation

True or False.

1. T F A medical chart is a legal document.

2. T F Information in a resident's chart may be shared with anyone who asks for it.

3. T F It is appropriate to chart care before it has been performed.

4. T F A nursing assistant should write his initials after each note he makes in the chart.

5. T F When documenting, use only facts.

6. T F If an error is made while document-ing, cross it out by drawing big circles through it.

7. T F Use accepted abbreviations and terms when documenting.

10. Describe the use of computers in documentation

Word Search.
Fill in each of the blanks and find your answers in the word search.

1. Computers can easily store information that can be _____ when needed.

2. Using a computer for charting is faster and more _____ than writing by hand.

3. Some facilities have a computer in every res-ident's _____.

4. Do not share personal _____ or _____ ID with anyone.

5. Do not access _____ e-mail or inappropriate _____ from work.

6. _____ privacy guidelines apply to computer use.

```
e k g a v s a d a i c g b c
g s j s f t y e a e f s n q
g l u n q i m v v b l g f y
v g e l k o h e m p q b o k
w p l n m e r i e c x p a r
r z i w h s d r o w s s a p
m q m a g g s t x b m e p w
j h n m t o n e w q b t i g
s g y l n z z r t j n y h b
q l a a k a l o g i n h q f
z m l i c c x o w z s y z e
w i a u y k a m d h u b w u
y e a s f k m f h s a i e b
j o n d f y q g y x v l v w
c e e s u z e m k w b t l o
k h n l q c w i j i z c g z
f n d h p r a v g x i m f n
l q y i k v g e u v f l m f
a g n c o m l r i z c j s s
k c u y l c y j r e s f z z
```

11. Explain the Minimum Data Set (MDS)

Multiple Choice.

1. The Minimum Data Set (MDS) was created to:
   a. Give facilities a structured, standardized approach to care
   b. Give facilities more flexibility in how care is performed
   c. Improve infection control in facilities
   d. Help train nursing assistants

2. Which of the following is NOT a time that a MDS would need to be completed for a resident?
   a. Within 14 days of admission
   b. At least once a year after the first MDS
   c. When there is a major change in a resi-dent's condition
   d. When a resident leaves the facility

3. What is the nursing assistant's role regarding the MDS?
   a. Completing the MDS for each resident
   b. Reminding the nurse when the MDS needs to be done
   c. Reporting on changes in residents' health that may trigger a needed assessment
   d. Deciding how to address problems discovered in the assessment

12. Describe how to observe and report accurately

True or False.

1. T F Any change in a resident's condition that is not serious does not need to be reported.

2. T F Nursing assistants may notice more changes in residents than other care team members because they spend the most time with residents.

3. T F Changes in a resident's condition that endanger residents should be reported right away.

4. T F Nursing assistants make decisions regarding residents' health.

5. T F Critical thinking for nursing assistants means the ability to make good observations.

6. T F A care plan is a written plan for each resident that outlines the steps and tasks needed to help the resident achieve his or her goals.

7. T F Care plans are created by nursing assistants.

8. T F Changes in a resident's weight do not need to be reported.

Fill in the Blank.

For each of the following, decide whether it is subjective data (the resident must tell you about it) or objective data (data you collect using your senses). Write "O" for objective or "S" for subjective.

1. _____ Red streaks on skin

2. _____ Swollen foot

3. _____ Nausea

4. _____ Itchy arm

5. _____ Dizziness

6. _____ Fever

7. _____ Vomiting

8. _____ Chest pain

Short Answer.

1. What is the nursing assistant's role in planning resident care?

   _____

   _____

   _____

   _____

   _____

   _____

   _____

   _____

2. For each of these four senses, list two observations that a nursing assistant might make using that sense.

   • Sight

   _____

   _____

   _____

   _____

   • Hearing

   _____

   _____

   _____

   _____

   • Smell

   _____

   _____

_____

_____

_____

- Touch

_____

_____

_____

_____

3. List three other ways to observe residents accurately.

_____

_____

_____

_____

_____

_____

4. List five signs and symptoms that should be reported immediately.

_____

_____

_____

_____

_____

_____

_____

13. Explain the nursing process

Matching.
Write the letter of the correct description beside each step of the nursing process.

a. In agreement with the resident, goals are set and a care plan is created to meet the resident's needs

b. A careful examination to see if goals were met or progress was achieved

c. Getting information from many sources to identify actual and potential problems

d. Putting the care plan into action; giving care

e. The identification of health problems after looking at all of the resident's needs

1. _____ Assessment

2. _____ Diagnosis

3. _____ Planning

4. _____ Implementation

5. _____ Evaluation

14. Discuss the nursing assistant's role in care planning and at care conferences

Multiple Choice.

1. The purpose of a care conference is:
   a. To train nursing assistants in new care skills
   b. To decide how to remove a resident from a facility
   c. To share and gather information about residents to develop a plan of care
   d. To orient new residents to the facility

2. What is the nursing assistant's role at a care conference?
   a. Keeping order at the meeting
   b. Sharing observations gathered from resident care
   c. Writing down the care plan
   d. Explaining the care plan to the resident and family

3. If a nursing assistant is not sure what to say at a care conference, she should
   a. Not attend the conference
   b. Attend the conference but not say anything
   c. Talk to the nurse before the conference to find out
   d. Ask other team members at the meeting what information to share

15. Describe incident reporting and recording

True or False.

1. T F It is okay to change the facts a little when writing an incident report.

2. T F Incident reports do not need to be made if the injury is a small one.

3. T F An incident is an accident, problem, or unexpected event that is not part of the normal routine of care.

4. T F An incident report should be completed as soon as possible after the incident occurs so that details are not forgotten.

5. T F The information in an incident report is available to the public.

6. T F Both facts and opinions are included in an incident report.

16. Explain proper telephone etiquette

Multiple Choice.

1. An example of proper telephone etiquette is:
   a. Immediately putting the caller on hold without asking
   b. Cheerfully identifying the facility to the caller
   c. Telling the caller, "Now is not a good time to call."
   d. Giving the caller any information she asks for about residents and staff

2. All of the following are reasons a nursing assistant should never give out any information regarding staff members or residents over the telephone EXCEPT:
   a. Nursing assistants will rarely have information about residents or staff.
   b. Problems such as domestic violence and stalking are increasing.
   c. All resident information is confidential.
   d. All staff information is confidential.

17. Describe the resident call system

Short Answer.

1. What is the purpose of the facility call system?

_____

_____

_____

_____

_____

_____

2. Why is answering a resident's call light promptly so important?

_____

_____

_____

_____

_____

_____

_____

18. Describe the nursing assistant's role in change-of-shift reports and "rounds"

Fill in the Blank.

1. Examples of information passed on to the next shift are _____ problems, complaints of _____, or a change in the ability to _____.

2. At start of shift reports, listen to important information about all of the _____ in the area.

3. Special information shared during a report may include new _____ and transfers or _____ from the facility.

4. Before the end of shift report, tell the nurses about such things as changes in

Name: _____

_____ or temperature and skin changes that could signal the start of a _____ _____ .

5. A method of reporting where staff members move from room to room and discuss each resident and the plan of care is called _____.

19. List the information found on an assignment sheet

Matching.

a. Exercises done to bring joints through a full range of movement

b. Tells whether a resident has an advance directive or not

c. Tasks that are done for residents every day

d. Advanced life support provided to a resident during an emergency

1. _____ Code

2. _____ Code status

3. _____ Range of motion

4. _____ Activities of daily living

20. Discuss how to organize your work and manage time

Crossword Puzzle.
Fill in each of the blanks below and use your answers to complete the crossword puzzle.

Across.

5. Do not be afraid to ask for _____.

6. Check to see if any residents require _____ help or care.

7. Making a schedule will help a nursing assistant be _____ about what can be done during the day.

8. Each facility will have its own _____ of events and care.

Down.

1. Write down anything important on the _____ sheet.

2. In order to complete assignments each day, a nursing assistant must learn to _____ his work.

3. A resident transferring to a _____ may change a nursing assistant's day.

4. _____ activities to be more efficient when possible.

7. Make _____ on all residents after receiving the day's assignment.

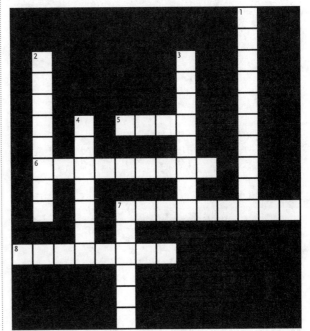

4
Communication Challenges

1. Review the key terms in Learning Objective 1 before completing the workbook exercises.

2. Identify communication guidelines for visual impairment

Word Search.
Fill in each of the blanks below and find your answers in the word search.

1. A(n) _____
    is a loss of function or ability.

2. _____ and
    _____ are two diseases that
    can cause visual impairment.

3. Do not _____
    a person with a visual impairment before
    speaking to him or her.

4. Make sure there is proper
    _____ in the room.

5. Do not _____.

6. Use the face of an imaginary
    _____
    to explain the position of objects.

7. If the resident has _____
    make sure they are clean and fit properly.

8. Do not move personal items or
    _____
    without the resident's permission.

9. Read _____ to the resident.

10. Do not play with or distract
    _____ _____.

11. Be _____
    and try to imagine what it feels like to not be
    able to see well.

```
e i y m t v j m o a e g u o
v c b u e i w b j d r l k w
u q o w t n s j j m u a x z
k h b i d f u i r s t u v l
s q z v c i g s z c i c d q
t n e m r i a p m i n o h b
e d z i w w t b s u r m c e
v k l j c o s e e i u a u t
x f f y g v r e h t f v o u
g u i d e d o g s t e q t b
g n i t h g i l j s a s l i
l c y x y j y r l m a p d z
c l o c k h e s l j n l m c
f n w w w c b y v r a c g e
```

3. Identify communication guidelines for hearing impairment

Multiple Choice.
Circle the letter of the correct answer.

1. All of the following are symptoms of hearing
    loss EXCEPT:
    a. Trouble hearing low-pitched noises
    b. Trouble hearing soft consonants
    c. Not understanding the meaning of words
    d. Being unable to hear people who are out-
        side of the room

2. Guidelines for communication with some-
    one who has a hearing impairment include:
    a. Exaggerate pronunciation of words.
    b. Cover the mouth with a hand while
        speaking.
    c. Chew gum while speaking.
    d. Use simple words and short sentences.

3. All of the following are ways to help people with a hearing impairment communicate more effectively EXCEPT:
   a. Hearing aids
   b. Lip reading
   c. Having a loud radio on in the room
   d. Picture cards

4. Explain defense mechanisms as methods of coping with stress

True or False.
Circle the "T" for true or the "F" for false for each of the following statements.

1. T F Defense mechanisms allow a person to release tension or cope with stress.

2. T F Repression means seeing feelings in others that are actually feelings within oneself.

3. T F Displacement means transferring a strong feeling to a less threatening object.

4. T F Defense mechanisms help a person to face the reasons a situation has occurred.

5. T F Denial is rejecting a thought or feeling.

6. T F Regression is making excuses to justify something.

5. List communication guidelines for anxiety or fear

Short Answer.
Answer each of the following questions in the space provided.

1. Define anxiety.

   _____

   _____

   _____

   _____

2. List four physical symptoms of anxiety.

   _____

   _____
   _____
   _____
   _____
   _____

3. List five guidelines for communicating with an anxious resident.

   _____

   _____

   _____

   _____

   _____

6. Discuss communication guidelines for depression

True or False.

1. T F Losses that a resident may be experiencing include the loss of a spouse, friends, and independence.

2. T F Depression can be managed, but it cannot be cured.

3. T F One behavior that is associated with depression is a lack of interest in activities.

4. T F Depression may be caused by a chemical imbalance.

5. T F Most people who are depressed could choose to be well if they wanted to.

6. T F It is never a good idea to touch a resident who is depressed.

7. T F Do not talk to adults as if they were children.

8. T F Depressed residents will never want to talk about their feelings.

9. T F Signs of depression should be reported right away.

7. Identify communication guidelines for anger

Fill in the Blank.
Fill in the correct word in each blank below.

1. _____ is a natural emotion that may be expressed by residents, their families, and staff.

2. Loss of _____ can cause a resident's anger.

3. Narrowed _____ and clenched or raised _____ are signs of anger.

4. Anger may also be expressed by withdrawing or being _____.

5. If a resident's anger requires more time from staff, a _____ _____ may be scheduled.

6. When dealing with an angry resident, try to find out what _____ the resident's anger.

7. Do not _____ with the resident.

8. Try to involve the resident in _____.

9. _____ means being confident in dealing with other people. _____ means expressing oneself in a way that humiliates or overpowers another person.

8. Identify communication guidelines for combative behavior

Multiple Choice.

1. Which of the following is probably NOT a cause of a resident's combative behavior?
   a. Personal reaction to a particular caregiver
   b. A disease affecting the brain
   c. Medication or changes in health
   d. Worsening of anger or frustration

2. A nursing assistant's responsibility when a resident becomes combative is to:
   a. Leave the resident alone.
   b. Tell the resident that he is upsetting everyone and needs to stop.
   c. Keep everyone safe.
   d. Threaten to restrain the resident if he doesn't calm down.

3. Under what circumstances may a nursing assistant hit a resident?
   a. Anytime a resident becomes combative
   b. If the resident threatens to hit the nursing assistant
   c. Only if the resident actually hits the nursing assistant
   d. Never

9. Identify communication guidelines for inappropriate sexual behavior

Crossword Puzzle.
Fill in each of the blanks below and use your answers to complete the crossword puzzle.

Across.

4. Nursing assistants must not _____ a resident's sexual behavior.

5. If a resident is engaging in a sexual act, the nursing assistant's role is to provide _____.

6. If a nursing assistant encounters an embarrassing situation, he should be calm and try to _____ the person.

8. Changes in the _____ may make a person unable to tell if behavior is improper.

9. Residents have the right to engage in mutually-agreed-upon _____ relationships.

Down.

1. Inappropriate sexual behavior makes the nursing assistant or others _____.

Name: _____

2. There is a _____
of sexual behavior in all age groups, including residents.

3. Inappropriate sexual behavior includes sexual _____ or comments.

7. Confused residents who have a
_____ or uncomfortable clothes
may appear to show inappropriate behavior.

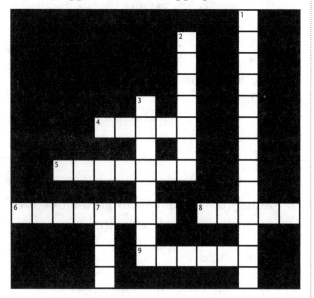

10. Identify communication guidelines for disorientation and confusion

Short Answer.

1. Define disorientation and confusion.

_____

_____

_____

_____

_____

_____

_____

2. List three things that a resident who is
oriented should be able to tell the nursing
assistant.

_____

_____

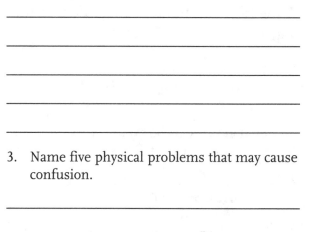

3. Name five physical problems that may cause
confusion.

_____

_____

_____

_____

_____

_____

4. What are three things a nursing assistant
can do to create a more comfortable environment for a resident who is confused?

_____

_____

_____

_____

_____

_____

_____

_____

5. How can a nursing assistant make tasks
easier for a person who is disoriented or
confused?

_____

_____

_____

_____

Name: _____

_____

_____

_____

11. Identify communication guidelines for the comatose resident

Multiple Choice.

1. All of the following are true of a coma EXCEPT:
   a. The person in a coma is in a state of unconsciousness.
   b. It usually occurs due to illness, a condition, or injury.
   c. A person in a coma cannot hear anything that is said in the room.
   d. A person in a coma cannot respond to a change in the environment.

2. Which of the following should a nursing assistant NOT do when caring for a resident who is in a coma?
   a. Hold personal conversations with others in the room.
   b. Introduce herself when entering the room.
   c. Explain each procedure she will be performing.
   d. Announce when she is leaving the room.

12. Identify communication guidelines for functional barriers

Fill in the Blank.

1. Some things that can interfere with the ability to speak include difficulty in _____, physical problems with the _____ or _____, or an artificial _____.

2. If a resident has difficulty breathing, never push the resident to _____.

3. Birth defects such as cleft _____ may make speech difficult.

4. Some residents who are _____ _____ will need an artificial airway.

5. A(n) _____ is a surgical opening made directly into the trachea.

6. Ask the resident to _____ _____ anything that is not understood.

7. Do not remove a resident's _____ for any reason.

8. Always report mouth sores and complaints of mouth pain as well as poorly fitting _____.

9. Be _____ to the resident's situation by imagining how it might feel to have a tube in the nose, mouth or throat.

5
Diversity and Human Needs and Development

1. Review the key terms in Learning Objective 1 before completing the workbook exercises

2. Explain health and wellness

Short Answer.
Answer each of the following questions in the space provided.

1. Define health and wellness.

_____

_____

_____

_____

_____

_____

_____

2. What is the focus of health?

_____

_____

_____

_____

_____

_____

3. For each of the five types of wellness, think of one thing that a nursing assistant can do to help residents achieve wellness in that area.

_____

_____

_____

_____

_____

_____

_____

_____

_____

_____

_____

_____

3. Explain the importance of holistic care

Multiple Choice.
Circle the letter of the correct answer.

1. Holistic care involves:
   a. Dividing a system into parts
   b. Caring for a person's physical needs
   c. Caring for a person's psychosocial needs
   d. Caring for the whole person

2. Which of the following is an example of a psychosocial need?
   a. Need for food
   b. Spirituality
   c. Need to be free from pain
   d. Need for shelter

3. Which of the following is a good example of giving holistic care to a resident?
   a. Asking a resident to talk about her day while giving her a bath
   b. Rushing a resident through dinner to get tasks done more quickly
   c. Choosing a resident's clothes for him so he doesn't have to worry about it
   d. Trying to convert a resident to the nursing assistant's religion

4. Identify basic human needs and discuss "Maslow's Hierarchy of Needs"

Fill in the Blank.
Fill in the correct word in each blank below.

1. A _____
   is something necessary for a person to survive and grow.

2. Residents need to feel as if they
   _____
   in their new home.

3. The first needs nursing assistants help residents meet are _____
   needs like food and water, rest and sleep.

4. Moving a person from her home into a facility can cause _____.

5. Residents may feel less of a sense of self-worth as they become
   _____ on others.

6. The highest need a person can achieve, according to Maslow, is _____
   _____.

5. Identify ways to accommodate cultural differences

True or False.
Circle the "T" for true or the "F" for false for each of the following statements.

1. T F A nursing assistant will not need an understanding of different cultures to care for residents.

2. T F Culture and background do not affect the way people behave when they are ill.

3. T F A nursing assistant should respond to new ideas with acceptance rather than prejudice.

4. T F People of all cultures tend to be embarrassed about discussing their health.

5. T F Ask residents and their friends and families about their traditions and customs to give better care.

6. T F If a resident does not understand the language the nursing assistant is speaking, the nursing assistant does not need to explain care procedures she is going to perform.

6. Discuss the role of the family in health care

Multiple Choice.

1. Which of the following is NOT an example of a family?
   a. Single parent with one or more children
   b. The staff and residents of the facility
   c. Unmarried couples of the same or opposite sex
   d. Divorced or widowed parents who have remarried and their children

2. When should staff become involved with family issues?
   a. Throughout the resident's stay in the facility
   b. Whenever the family has disagreements
   c. When there is concern about a resident's safety around family members
   d. Never

3. Which of the following is NOT a way that families help support their loved ones who are residents?
   a. Abusing the resident
   b. Helping make care decisions
   c. Taking residents out for walks
   d. Joining residents for activities or outside functions

4. When residents have visitors, a nursing assistant should:
   a. Do everything possible to help the resident prepare for the visit.
   b. Ignore the visitors.
   c. Tell the resident's family funny stories about him.
   d. Watch the family closely to make sure the resident is not abused during the visit.

7. Explain how to meet emotional needs of residents and their families

Crossword Puzzle.
Fill in each of the blanks below and use your answers to complete the crossword puzzle.

Across.

3. When residents come to a nursing assistant with problems or needs, he should listen closely and not

   _____.

5. Residents and families may go to a nursing assistant during a(n)

   _____

   crisis.

8. When families ask questions regarding a resident's _____,
   treatments, and therapies, refer them to the nurse.

9. Respond to worry or fear with a(n)

   _____

   message.

10. Nursing assistants may be the person residents turn to when they feel fear,

    _____ or stress.

Down.

1. It is important for a nursing assistant to maintain _____
   boundaries with residents and their families.

2. Nursing assistants are the

   _____

   caregivers for their residents.

4. Offer support and

   _____.

6. Do not respond with _____.

7. If a resident dies, her family may seek a nursing assistant out for

   _____ or

   to talk.

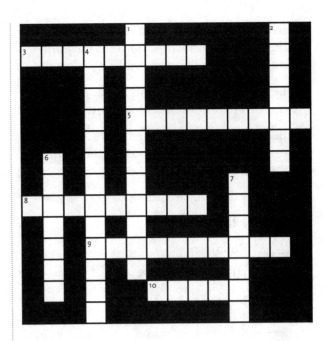

8. Explain ways to help residents with their spiritual needs

True or False.

1. T F A resident's religious items must be handled carefully.

2. T F Respecting religious beliefs includes telling Muslim residents about Christianity.

3. T F Spiritual needs are different for each person.

4. T F Some people consider themselves spiritual but do not believe in a higher power.

5. T F Residents who do not believe in God will not feel as strongly as residents who do.

Matching.
Write the letter of the correct description beside each religious faith.

a. The Five Pillars of this religion include ritual prayer five times daily and donations to the poor and needy

b. May be baptized and take communion

c. Believe that they do not know or cannot know if God exists

Name: _____

d. Believe that a person can reach Nirvana, the highest spiritual plane, after traveling through birth, life, and death

e. Believe that actions in this life and past lives can determine one's destiny in future lives

f. Believe that God gave them laws and commandments through Moses in the form of the Torah

g. Actively deny the existence of God

1. ____ Islam

2. ____ Buddhism

3. ____ Hinduism

4. ____ Judaism

5. ____ Atheist

6. ____ Christianity

7. ____ Agnostic

9. Identify ways to accommodate sexual needs

True or False.

1. T F Most residents do not have sexual needs.

2. T F Sexual identity does not play a very important role in a person's life.

3. T F A transsexual person wishes to be accepted by society as a member of the opposite sex.

4. T F Elderly people are not interested in sex.

5. T F Illness may affect how a resident expresses himself sexually.

6. T F Any expression of sexuality by older people is either disgusting or cute.

7. T F If a nursing assistant encounters a resident engaging in a sexual activity, she should provide privacy.

8. T F Residents have the right to choose how to express themselves sexually.

9. T F If a nursing assistant sees a resident being sexually abused, she should not report it because it might embarrass the resident.

Short Answer.

1. Gilda and Samantha both live in a nursing home. Gilda is widowed and Samantha has never been married. They met when Gilda was admitted six months ago. Gilda and Samantha have been sitting at the same table to eat their meals since Gilda moved in. Recently they have started spending time watching TV and playing cards in the day room together. Yesterday they took a walk outside. Linda, a nursing assistant, was gazing out the window and noticed them holding hands. Then she saw them stop behind the building and share a quick kiss. What are some responses that would respect Samantha and Gilda's dignity and rights?

_____

_____

_____

_____

_____

_____

_____

2. Mr. Ramirez has a private room. His wife lives quite a distance away and only visits once every two weeks. The last time she visited, she requested a dinner tray and asked for both meals to be brought to his room. When Linda went to his room to deliver the meals, the door was shut. She walked in without knocking, and found them kissing each other in bed. She quickly exited the room, and almost dropped the food on her way out. What could Linda have done differently? What should she do now that there has been an embarrassing moment?

_____

_____

_____

_____

_____

Name: _____

_____

_____

_____

3. List and describe four terms that define sexual identity.

_____

_____

_____

_____

_____

_____

_____

_____

4. What are two reasons for a lack of sexual expression in nursing homes?

_____

_____

_____

_____

_____

5. List four ways to help residents with their sexual needs.

_____

_____

_____

_____

_____

_____

_____

_____

10. Describe the stages of human growth and development

Fill in the Blank.

1. _____refers to physical changes that can be measured.

2. _____ means the emotional, social and physical changes that occur in a person's life.

3. _____ development is the process of gaining an ability to do such things as walking, drawing, and grasping.

4. _____development is the process of children forming a sense of right and wrong.

5. _____ development focuses on how children think and learn.

6. _____ development is the process of learning to relate to other people.

7. _____ development has to do with the reproductive changes that occur when young people reach puberty.

Multiple Choice.

1. In which stage of development is playing dress-up in parents' clothing common?
    a. Toddler
    b. Pre-school
    c. Adolescence
    d. Infancy

2. Both genders become fully sexually mature during:
    a. School-age
    b. Adolescence
    c. Middle adulthood
    d. Late adulthood

3. Decisions about education, employment, and marriage often occur during this stage:
    a. Young adulthood
    b. Middle adulthood
    c. Late adulthood
    d. Adolescence

4. All of the following are true of late adulthood EXCEPT:
   a. Couples may travel more to see friends,
      family, and children.
   b. Mobility can become limited.
   c. People no longer need to stay connected
      to others.
   d. People may retire from their jobs.

11. Discuss stereotypes of the elderly

Multiple Choice.

1. A biased generalization based on false
   beliefs about a group is:
   a. Stereotyping
   b. Ageism
   c. Opinions
   d. Discrimination

2. All of the following are usually bases for ste-
   reotypes about a group EXCEPT:
   a. Opinions
   b. Distorted ideas
   c. Getting to know individuals of a particu-
      lar group
   d. Television and movies

3. Most older people:
   a. Do not like to leave home
   b. Are active and have many interests
   c. Cannot manage their money
   d. Are ill and dependent

12. Discuss developmental disabilities

True or False.

1. T F Developmental disabilities are present
         at birth or emerge during childhood.

2. T F Developmental disabilities can be
         cured.

3. T F Developmental disabilities cause dif-
         ficulty with language, learning, and
         self-care.

4. T F The most common developmental
         disability is autism.

5. T F People with developmental disabili-
         ties prefer to be treated like children.

Name: _____

6
Infection Control

1. Review the **key terms** in Learning Objective 1 before completing the workbook exercises

2. Define "infection control" and discuss types of infections

Matching.
Write the letter of the correct definition beside each term listed at right.

a. A tiny living thing not visible without a microscope

b. Infection that moves throughout the body

c. The body's ability to prevent infection and disease

d. Harmful microorganism that causes disease

e. Infection that is limited to one area of the body

f. Infection acquired in a hospital

g. Being infected a second time with an infection.

h. Occurs when a pathogen is spread from one person to another

i. Set of methods used to control and prevent the spread of disease

j. Infection associated with various healthcare settings, such as long-term care facilities and ambulatory settings

1. _____   Communicable disease

2. _____   Healthcare-associated infection (HAI)

3. _____   Infection control

4. _____   Localized infection

5. _____   Microorganism

6. _____   Nosocomial infection

7. _____   Pathogen

8. _____   Reinfection

9. _____   Resistance

10. _____   Systemic infection

3. Discuss terms related to infection control

True or False.
Circle the "T" for true or the "F" for false for each of the following statements.

1. T F   Sterilization means all microorganisms are destroyed, including pathogens and spores.

2. T F   Medical asepsis means that a facility is completely free from microorganisms.

3. T F   You must wash your hands before entering a clean utility room.

4. T F   Transmission is the process of removing pathogens.

5. T F   An object can be called "clean" if it has not been contaminated with pathogens.

6. T F   Hard-shelled microorganisms called spores are killed by disinfection.

7. T F   Clean and dirty equipment, linen, and supplies are stored in the same utility room.

4. Describe the chain of infection

Short Answer.
Answer each of the following questions in the space provided.

Name: _____

1. What does the chain of infection describe?

_____

_____

_____

_____

_____

2. How many links in the chain of infection must be broken for infection to be prevented?

_____

_____

_____

3. List the links of the chain of infection.

_____

_____

_____

_____

_____

_____

_____

5. Explain why the elderly are at a higher risk for infection

Multiple Choice.
Circle the letter of the correct answer.

1. One reason that older people are at a greater risk for acquiring infections is:
   a. Their immune systems become stronger.
   b. They are hospitalized more often.
   c. Elderly people recover more quickly from illness.
   d. Infections are less dangerous in older people.

2. All of the following are factors associated with aging that increase danger of infection EXCEPT:
   a. Thinning skin
   b. Limited mobility
   c. Increased circulation
   d. Use of catheters and other tubing

3. All of the following may be causes of malnutrition and dehydration EXCEPT:
   a. Too much fluid in the body
   b. Lack of thirst and appetite
   c. Illness
   d. Medication

6. Describe the Centers for Disease Control and Prevention (CDC) and explain Standard Precautions

Fill in the Blank.
Fill in the correct word in each blank below.

1. The abbreviation for the government agency that promotes public health and safety and attempts to control and prevent disease:

   _____.

2. The two levels of precautions in the infection control system recommended by the CDC are Standard Precautions and

   _____

   _____ _____.

3. Standard Precautions means treating all blood, body fluids, non-intact skin and mucous membranes as if they were

   _____.

4. You cannot tell by looking at residents or their charts if they have a(n)

   _____ disease.

5. Wear a _____
   and protective _____ if you may come into contact with splashing or spraying body fluids.

6. Razor blades and other sharps should be disposed of in a _____ container.

7. Never transfer _____
   items or any kind of _____
   from one room to another.

8. Never place _____
   items on the overbed table.

9. When cleaning anything, move from the
    _____ to the
    _____ area.

7. Define "hand hygiene" and identify when to wash hands

True or False.

1. T F   Handwashing is the single most
           important method to reduce the
           spread of infection.

2. T F   Bacteria can be removed from false
           nails with thorough handwashing.

3. T F   Use of unscented lotions reduces risk
           of broken skin on hands.

4. T F   A nursing assistant must wash her
           hands every time she removes her
           gloves.

5. T F   A nursing assistant must wash his
           hands if he blows his nose.

6. T F   A nursing assistant does not need
           to wash her hands before obtaining
           clean linen from a cart.

7. T F   Use friction for no more than five
           seconds while washing hands.

8. T F   Using alcohol-based hand rubs mean
           that nursing assistants never have to
           wash their hands.

8. Discuss the use of personal protective equipment (PPE) in facilities

True or False.

1. T F   PPE is not important in preventing
           transmission of disease.

2. T F   The type of PPE a nursing assistant
           wears depends on what kind of expo-
           sure may be encountered.

3. T F   Gowns have to be worn if you may
           come into contact with splashing or
           spraying blood or body fluids.

4. T F   Gowns do not need to be changed if
           they become soiled or wet.

5. T F   Masks can prevent microorganisms
           from being inhaled.

6. T F   Masks should fit snugly over the nose
           and mouth.

7. T F   Special PPE will be required for a
           resident with tuberculosis.

8. T F   It does not matter in what order PPE
           is put on or removed.

Fill in the Blank.
Mark an "X" next to the tasks that require you to wear gloves.

1. ____   Contact with body fluids

2. ____   Hanging laundry

3. ____   When you may touch blood

4. ____   Brushing a resident's hair

5. ____   Assisting with perineal care

6. ____   Giving a massage to a resident with
           acne on his back

7. ____   Hugging residents

8. ____   Shaving a resident

9. List guidelines for handling linen and equipment

Crossword Puzzle.
Fill in each of the blanks below and use your answers to complete the crossword puzzle.

Across.

2. Dispose of all _____ _____
    equipment properly.

4. Facilities handle storage and disposal of lin-
    ens and equipment by following guidelines
    set by the _____.

5. Do not touch the inside of any
    _____ container.

7. Do not _____
    dirty linen or clothes.

8. Facilities have separate areas for clean and
    _____ items.

9. Wear _____
    when handling and processing soiled linens.

Name: _____

Down.

1. There will be containers for special disposal of _____ waste.

3. All sharps must be placed in puncture-proof _____ containers.

6. Fold or roll linen so that the dirtiest area is _____.

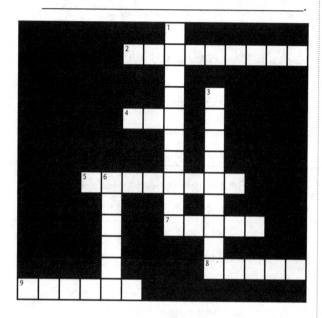

10. Explain how to handle spills

Short Answer.

1. Why are spills in a facility dangerous?

_____

_____

_____

_____

2. What kind of solution should be used to clean up a spill?

_____

_____

_____

_____

3. If a nursing assistant spills a substance on her body, what should she do?

_____

_____

_____

_____

11. Discuss Transmission-Based Precautions

Fill in the Blank.
Fill in each blank with the correct type of isolation precaution: "A" for Airborne, "D" for Droplet, or "C" for Contact.

1. ____ These are used when the disease-causing microorganism only travels short distances after being expelled.

2. ____ Transmission of a microorganism can occur with direct contact, for example, a nursing assistant bathing a resident.

3. ____ These precautions reduce the risk of spreading tuberculosis.

4. ____ Microorganisms can be spread by talking, singing, or sneezing.

5. ____ Diseases can be transmitted through the air over long distances.

6. ____ Infection can be spread by touching contaminated personal items.

12. Describe care of the resident in an isolation unit

Short Answer.

1. Why is it important to spend as much time as possible with a resident who is in isolation?

_____

_____

_____

_____

_____

2. List five ways to help a resident in isolation feel connected to the outside world.

Name: _____

_____

_____

_____

_____

_____

_____

_____

3. List four of the steps involved in setting up an isolation unit.

_____

_____

_____

_____

_____

_____

13. Explain OSHA's Bloodborne Pathogen Standard

Word Search.
Fill in each of the blanks and find your answers in the word search.

1. _____
   is the government agency that regulates the safety of workers in the U.S.

2. The _____
   _____
   Standard is the law that requires healthcare facilities to protect employees from bloodborne health hazards.

3. A(n) _____
   _____ is
   when an employee is exposed to infectious blood or material.

4. A(n) _____
   _____ plan
   identifies what is supposed to be done if anyone is exposed to infectious waste.

5. Infection can be spread by having accidental contact with contaminated blood or body fluids, skin, _____
   or other sharp objects, or
   _____
   supplies or equipment.

6. The employer is responsible for providing a free _____ _____
   vaccine to all employees after hire.

```
c  i  l  b  f  l  j  t  y  n  k  v  l  h
l  a  o  l  k  o  y  n  b  q  s  a  g  c
m  g  b  o  m  r  c  e  g  z  k  p  h  j
u  w  k  o  q  t  q  d  u  k  m  t  v  m
s  t  v  d  v  n  c  i  o  v  q  j  x  q
g  v  a  b  b  o  q  c  t  a  w  e  o  w
t  k  r  o  i  c  l  n  m  b  k  n  m  x
u  w  b  r  j  e  y  i  y  n  x  s  y  a
o  l  g  n  e  r  y  e  e  b  c  o  k  f
d  s  d  e  t  u  c  r  a  b  k  b  d  h
h  v  h  p  x  s  c  u  z  t  k  s  c  p
c  t  a  a  x  o  a  s  r  w  k  i  a  l
s  s  z  t  w  p  s  o  l  b  n  t  e  d
a  p  a  h  f  x  o  p  g  w  t  i  d  a
b  y  r  o  o  e  h  x  u  h  c  t  c  q
i  m  d  g  w  u  w  e  c  i  o  a  g  g
n  m  s  e  l  d  e  e  n  e  p  p  a  k
j  c  o  n  t  a  m  i  n  a  t  e  d  h
l  b  a  t  e  r  t  d  p  y  s  h  y  a
h  d  u  m  e  t  l  l  z  u  g  p  w  c
```

14. Discuss two important bloodborne diseases

Multiple Choice.

1. How does the HIV virus cause the body to be unable to fight infection?
   a. Causes cirrhosis
   b. Causes liver cancer
   c. Damages the immune system
   d. Poisons the blood

2. HIV can be spread by all of the following EXCEPT:
   a. Sexual contact
   b. Use of infected needles
   c. Hugging
   d. Passing to fetus from mother

3. Hepatitis ___ and ___ are bloodborne diseases that can cause death.
   a. A and B
   b. B and C
   c. C and D
   d. A and C

4. Ways to prevent hepatitis B include all of the
following EXCEPT:
   a. Use proper PPE on the job.
   b. Handle needles and other sharps carefully.
   c. Get the vaccine for hepatitis B when it is
offered.
   d. Share a resident's razor or toothbrush
with another resident.

15. Discuss MRSA, VRE, and C. *difficile*

True or False.

1. T F   Multidrug-resistant organisms
(MDROs) are not a serious problem
in healthcare facilities.

2. T F   MRSA is mostly spread by direct
physical contact.

3. T F   The most important way to control
MRSA and VRE is through proper
hand hygiene.

4. T F   *Enterococcus* often causes problems in
healthy people.

5. T F   VRE is easily controlled with antibiotics.

6. T F   Residents with MRSA or VRE should
not be around other people or participate in any activities.

7. T F   Overuse of antibiotics may alter the
normal intestinal flora and increase
the risk of developing *C. difficile.*

8. T F   There is no test that can diagnose *C.
difficile.*

Name: _____

7
Safety and Body Mechanics

1. Review the key terms in Learning Objective 1 before completing the workbook exercises

2. List common accidents in facilities and ways to prevent them

True or False.
Circle the "T" for true or the "F" for false for each of the following statements.

1. T F An important way to help prevent falls is to respond to call lights promptly.

2. T F Loose-fitting clothing and pants that are too long are the best types of clothing to prevent falls.

3. T F A nursing assistant must identify each resident before providing care or serving food.

4. T F Demented or confused residents do not have to be identified since they do not understand who they are anyway.

5. T F Burns can cause a rapid deterioration in a resident's condition.

6. T F In order to prevent burns, water temperature of a bath should be over 128°F.

7. T F Liquids can cause burns.

8. T F A disoriented resident may eat hair care products or flowers.

9. T F To aid in poison prevention, serve residents foods that are over a month old.

10. T F Sitting up straight while eating helps prevent choking.

11. T F Large pieces of food are less likely to cause choking.

12. T F Protecting arms and legs while moving residents helps prevent injury.

13. T F If a nursing assistant needs help lifting a resident, but nobody is around, she should go ahead and lift the resident anyway.

14. T F After an eye splash, if no eye wash station is available, rinse the eye immediately with water.

3. Explain the Material Safety Data Sheet (MSDS)

Short Answer.
Answer each of the following questions in the space provided.

1. List five examples of information that is found on an MSDS.

_____

_____

_____

_____

_____

_____

_____

2. What are two things that a nursing assistant must know about the MSDS?

_____

_____

_____

_____

_____

4. Describe safety guidelines for sharps and biohazard containers

Fill in the Blank.
Fill in the correct word in each blank below.

1. Always wear _____ when disposing of infectious waste.

2. It is important to keep _____ above the opening of a biohazard container.

3. When touching a sharps container, touch the _____ of the container only.

4. Sharps containers should be replaced when they are _____ full or following facility policy.

5. Biohazard containers are used to dispose of anything contaminated with infectious waste except for anything _____.

5. Explain the principles of body mechanics and apply them to daily activities

Matching.
Write the letter of the correct definition beside each term.

a. Foundation that supports an object

b. The point in the body where the most weight is concentrated

c. When the two sides of the body are mirror images of each other

d. The way the parts of the body work together when a person moves

e. Important problems that nursing assistants face

1. _____ Back and body strain and injury

2. _____ Body mechanics

3. _____ Alignment

4. _____ Base of support

5. _____ Center of gravity

Short Answer.

1. List five activities in a facility that require moving or lifting something.

_____
_____
_____
_____
_____
_____
_____
_____
_____

2. List eight ways to use proper body mechanics on the job.

_____
_____
_____
_____
_____
_____
_____
_____
_____
_____
_____
_____

6. Define two types of restraints and discuss problems associated with restraints

Multiple Choice.
Circle the letter of the correct answer.

1. Why has the use of restraints in facilities been restricted?
   a. Restraints are too expensive.
   b. Restraint usage was abused by caregivers.
   c. Training nursing assistants to use restraints is too difficult.
   d. Nursing assistants do not have time to monitor residents who are restrained.

2. When may restraints be used?
    a. For staff convenience
    b. With a doctor's order
    c. To discipline residents
    d. Whenever staff wants to use them

3. All of the following are potential negative effects of restraint use EXCEPT:
    a. Increased blood circulation
    b. Pressure sores
    c. Loss of self-esteem
    d. Death

7. Define the terms "restraint free" and "restraint alternatives" and list examples of restraint alternatives

Word Search.
Fill in each of the blanks below and find your answers in the word search.

```
i s p h v r a z c d f c x b
c e x k d o v v k c f a c q
t v o h t p w a n d e r p q
i i d r v t c e h z u e f a
k t c x l y g j s n o g i c
r a q a r i o x m u s i c k
d n m h d t o n e l y v z c
d r d s a k h o d a q e k r
s e p k m p m g r e j r e v
n t d o x r n p r x d s n v
t l e b m b a x g e t d m s
t a d s l f i l n r e u n j
s t h g i l l l a c p s k x
o n o c m o c i c i b g h j
y i r y z r n q t s c v r n
v a q h t t f j q e l o x g
s r l s f p k j b m h f s g
x t f r a o d i s j b m n n
k s e o f l k x h p s b x v
i e p e n w k w p i y s x f
j r r p r p h d g u i g i d
```

1. _____ _____
    care means that restraints are not kept or used for any reason.

2. Creative ideas that help avoid the use of restraints are called _____
    _____.

3. Answer _____
    _____
    immediately.

4. Add more _____
    into the care plan.

5. Let confused residents
    _____
    in designated safe areas.

6. Increase visits and _____
    interaction.

7. Increase number of familiar
    _____.

8. Decrease the _____
    level.

9. Use soothing _____.

10. Bed or body _____
    alert staff when residents attempt to leave the bed or chair.

8. Describe beginning and ending steps in care procedures

Short Answer.

1. Why should a nursing assistant identify herself and the resident before performing care?

    _____
    _____
    _____
    _____
    _____
    _____
    _____
    _____
    _____
    _____
    _____
    _____

2. Why is it important for a nursing assistant to provide for the resident's privacy each time before giving care?

_____

_____

_____

_____

_____

_____

3. Why is it important to place the call light within the resident's reach before leaving the room?

_____

_____

_____

_____

_____

4. Why should a nursing assistant report any changes in the resident to the nurse? Why should she document the procedure properly after giving care?

_____

_____

_____

_____

_____

_____

_____

_____

9. Identify what must be done if a restraint is ordered

Crossword Puzzle.
Fill in each of the blanks below and use your answers to complete the crossword puzzle.

Across.

4. After restraints are removed, offer the resident a trip to the

_____ or a

change of incontinent briefs.

5. Place your hand in a _____

_____ between the resident and the restraint to ensure that the device fits properly and is comfortable.

8. Restraints must be removed every

_____ hours or more often if needed.

9. Check on the resident every

_____ minutes for most restraints.

Down.

1. Place the _____

_____ within reach of the resident at all times.

2. A(n) _____

_____ is a quick-release knot used to tie restraints so that they can be removed quickly when needed.

3. Make sure there is a written

_____

_____ for a restraint before applying one.

6. Never tie the restraints to

_____

_____ ;

only tie to movable part of a bed frame.

7. Check the area around the restraint for

_____ ,

or blue-tinged skin.

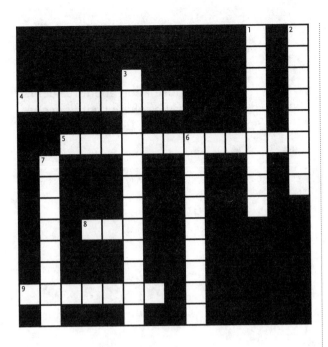

10. List safety guidelines for oxygen use

True or False.

1. T F Nursing assistants turn off and adjust oxygen levels.

2. T F Oxygen is a dangerous fire hazard.

3. T F Smoking should not be allowed anywhere around oxygen equipment.

4. T F Fire hazards that should be removed from residents' rooms include electric razors, hair dryers, and radios.

5. T F Combustion means easily ignited and capable of burning.

6. T F It is okay to use lighters and matches around oxygen.

7. T F Alcohol and nail polish remover are flammable liquids.

8. T F Wool and nylon clothing is safe for residents using oxygen.

11. Identify safety guidelines for intravenous (IV) lines

Fill in the Blank.

1. "IV" is an abbreviation for

_____,

or into a vein.

2. A resident with an IV is receiving

_____,

nutrition, or _____

through a vein.

3. A nursing assistant should always wear

_____

if she has to touch the IV area.

4. Do not take resident's _____

_____ in an arm with an IV.

5. Do not leave the tubing _____.

6. Do not disconnect the IV from the

_____ or turn off the

_____.

7. Report to the nurse if the needle or

_____ has fallen out.

8. Report to the nurse if

_____

appears in the tubing.

9. Report if the resident complains of

_____

or has difficulty _____.

10. Residents who have IVs have the right to freedom of _____.

12. Discuss fire safety and explain the "RACE" and "PASS" acronyms

Short Answer.

1. What are the three things needed for a fire to occur?

_____

_____

_____

_____

_____

2. List five potential causes of fire in facilities.

_____

_____

_____

_____

Name: _____

_____
_____
_____

3. Fill in the words for the following acronyms:

R _____

A _____

C _____

E _____

P _____

A _____

S _____

S _____

4. List four general procedures to follow in case of a fire.

_____
_____
_____
_____
_____
_____
_____

13. List general safety steps to protect yourself and residents in a facility

True or False.

1. T F   Living or working in a facility never puts a person at risk of crime.

2. T F   Very few people go in and out of a facility during the day.

3. T F   It is best to watch for suspicious behavior and report it immediately.

4. T F   It is a good idea for a nursing assistant to take valuables to work so that he can keep an eye on them.

5. T F   A nursing assistant should not leave a resident alone with a visitor or staff member who makes her uneasy.

6. T F   Personal information about residents and staff may be shared with anyone who asks.

8

Emergency Care, First Aid, and Disasters

1. Review the key terms in Learning Objective 1 before completing the workbook exercises

2. Demonstrate how to respond to medical emergencies

Short Answer.
Answer each of the following questions in the space provided.

1. What are the two types of PPE a nursing assistant should always have with him in case of an emergency?

_____

_____

_____

2. When would a face mask be used?

_____

_____

_____

_____

3. Why is it a good idea to carry two sets of gloves?

_____

_____

_____

_____

Multiple Choice.
Circle the letter of the correct answer.

1. All of the following are signs of a serious medical emergency EXCEPT:
   a. The person is conscious.
   b. The person is not breathing.
   c. The person has no pulse.
   d. The person is bleeding severely.

2. All of the following information should be included in an incident report EXCEPT:
   a. Signs and symptoms observed
   b. Actions taken
   c. The time at which a person becomes unconscious
   d. What the nursing assistant thinks happened to the person

3. Describe basic CPR and demonstrate knowledge of first aid procedures

Word Search.
Fill in each of the blanks below and find your answers in the word search.

1. When breathing stops, it is called _____ arrest.

2. When the heart stops, it is called _____ arrest.

3. _____
   _____,
   or _____,
   refers to medical procedures used when the heart or lungs have stopped working; it is used until medical help arrives.

4. CPR must be started immediately to prevent or minimize

   _____ _____.

5. Brain damage can occur within _____ to _____ minutes after the heart stops beating and breathing stops.

6. Only properly _____ people should perform CPR.

7. Performing CPR incorrectly can _____ _____ a person.

Name: _____

8. _____ _____ is the care given by the first people to respond to an emergency.

```
r t x c j f l g j l i b l t
c c v a m l p a h h j v r a
z x u r v g h p t t i d l a
u d o d q h u g q y x z k e
e l h i y v x d c i p b p b
o t w o q e g n e b r g y b
g k o p f z c v r a c u b z
j s i u b t a d i q j h o e
v g r l c a i n z r w k z f
l o v m o s d z x k w o u o
w y r o t a r i p s e r j i
z f v n m j a d d y t l v p
n i o a l d c i g h n p c s
b n g r u i j i e i e v g y
g e z y w d z r d o q z a q
t c q r f z i q o w u y l c
v c p e f n a x z d q j j l
c r w s j e j n e f j f x o
f l m u q a f n o g v z d f
f i r s t a i d y z i d y t
t e w c z a g o w d q h c b
c n a i r b b a t h l a s c
l x g t u p l w w r y g g b
e m a a x r c c e l b e n c
j t o t t g v h d v h s p i
i d s i x a l a d a q c i l
s c y o a v o b g q v p v n
r b w n j k e t l i y x o f
```

True or False.

Circle the "T" for true or the "F" for false for each of the following statements.

1. T F A nursing assistant can only initiate CPR if he is trained and authorized to do so.

2. T F To check a person's airway, tilt the head back slightly to open it.

3. T F A person in shock should sit upright until symptoms improve.

4. T F After notifying the nurse, the first step a nursing assistant should take when trying to control bleeding is to put on gloves.

5. T F When blood seeps through a pad that is being used to control bleeding, it should be removed and replaced with a clean pad.

6. T F Applying water to a serious burn may cause infection.

7. T F The medical term for vomiting is epistaxis.

8. T F Insulin reaction results from too much insulin or too little food.

9. T F Diabetic ketoacidosis may be caused by undiagnosed diabetes.

10. T F The medical term for a heart attack is transient ischemic attack (TIA).

Matching.

For each sign or symptom or response described below, write the letter of the emergency it applies to.

1. ____ Signs of this include pale or cyanotic skin, staring, increased pulse and respiration rates, decreased blood pressure, and extreme thirst.

2. ____ Hold a thick sterile pad directly on the wound.

3. ____ Signs of this include severe pain in the chest, anxiety, and heartburn or indigestion.

4. ____ Give abdominal thrusts until the object is pushed out or the person loses consciousness.

5. ____ Apply firm pressure over the bridge of the nose if this occurs.

6. ____ Never use any kind of ointment, salve, or grease on this.

7. ____ If a person is sitting, have her bend forward and place her head between her knees.

8. ____ Signs of this include loss of consciousness, loss of bowel and bladder control, and blurred vision.

9. ____ Do not try to stop this or hold the person down.

10. ____ Sweet or fruity breath is a symptom.

11. ____ If this occurs, it is a good idea to give the person a lump of sugar, candy, or a glass of orange juice immediately.

Name: _____

12. _____ Talk to the resident soothingly and give oral care.

13. _____ Signs of this include sudden collapse, vomiting, and heavy, difficult breathing.

a. Bleeding

b. Burns

c. Choking

d. Diabetic ketoacidosis

e. Fainting

f. Insulin reaction

g. Myocardial infarction

h. Nosebleed

i. Poisoning

j. Seizure

k. Shock

l. Stroke

m. Vomiting

4. Explain the nursing assistant's role on a code team

Fill in the Blank.
Fill in the correct word in each blank below.

1. Facilities use codes to inform staff of

   _____

   without alarming residents and visitors.

2. "Code Red" usually means

   _____,

   and "Code Blue" usually means

   _____

   _____.

3. The _____

   _____ is the

   team chosen for a shift to respond in case of a resident emergency.

4. Staff on the code team may be asked to get a special _____ or other emergency equipment.

5. Nursing assistants may be asked to do

   _____

   _____ during CPR.

6. Respond to codes after any residents you are caring for are _____.

5. Describe guidelines for responding to disasters

Short Answer.

1. What kinds of disasters are most likely to occur in your area?

   _____

   _____

   _____

   _____

   _____

   _____

   _____

2. Describe the way nursing assistants should respond to disasters.

   _____

   _____

   _____

   _____

   _____

9
Admission, Transfer, Discharge, and Physical Exams

1. Review the key terms in Learning Objective 1 before completing the workbook exercises

2. List factors for families in choosing a facility

Short Answer.
Answer each of the following questions in the space provided.

1. What are three sources of information that families may use to guide them in choosing a facility for a loved one?

_____

_____

_____

_____

_____

2. Why do you think family members ask so many questions before deciding on a facility?

_____

_____

_____

_____

_____

_____

_____

3. Explain the nursing assistant's role in the emotional adjustment of a new resident

Scenario.
Read the following scenario and answer the questions that follow.

New resident Suki Lee is having a hard time. She mostly cries in her room and refuses to par-

ticipate in any activity. Nursing assistant Stewart Johnson stops by her room to take her blood pressure. When he sees her crying by the window, he sighs loudly and rolls his eyes. "You're lucky I'm here," he says. "Nobody else knows how to deal with overly emotional residents."

He continues, "In fact, last week the resident in room 102 couldn't stop crying when he found out he has colon cancer. I was the only one he would talk to."

Ms. Lee continues to cry softly while he takes her blood pressure. "I don't know why you're so sad," he says. "I'd be happy if I could be somewhere where I got all my meals cooked and my room cleaned. Plus, there's lots of other old folks here to talk to."

He leaves her room and realizes he forgot to note her blood pressure. Not wanting to deal with her again, he thinks for a moment and writes down some numbers.

1. Name seven things Stewart could have done to take better care of Ms. Lee.

_____

_____

_____

_____

_____

_____

_____

_____

_____

_____

_____

_____

_____

_____

Name: _____

2. List five reasons that moving into a facility is a big emotional adjustment for new residents.

_____

_____

_____

_____

_____

_____

4. Describe the nursing assistant's role in the admission process

True or False.
Circle the "T" for true or the "F" for false for each of the following statements.

1. T F It is not important to give a new resident a good first impression of the staff and the facility.

2. T F Family and friends are a good source of information for a resident's personal preferences, history, and routines.

3. T F A new resident's admission pack may include soap, a bedpan, a pitcher and a cup.

4. T F It is better to wait until the resident has already arrived to start preparing her room.

5. T F The resident should not feel as if he is an inconvenience; he should feel welcome and wanted.

6. T F It is important to introduce new residents to other residents and staff members.

7. T F Baseline measurements are taken six months after admission to a facility.

8. T F Changes in residents' weight do not need to be reported.

9. T F There is no way to measure the weight or height of a resident who cannot get out of bed.

5. Explain the nursing assistant's role during an in-house transfer of a resident

Word Search.
Fill in each of the blanks on the following page and find your answers in the word search.

1. Residents may need to be transferred to a unit that offers more

_____ care.

2. _____ is always hard. This may be especially true if the resident has a(n) _____ or his condition has

_____.

3. Nursing assistants should try to make the transfer as _____ as possible for residents.

4. Residents have the right to be

_____

of any room or roommate change.

5. At the new unit, _____ the resident to everyone.

6. If a nursing assistant _____ the resident's belongings, she should do it carefully.

7. When leaving the resident's room, report to the _____ in charge of the resident.

```
p  l  i  f  s  w  t  x  b  w  f  k  y  g
z  s  c  r  m  n  e  u  p  i  f  a  a  b
e  u  h  s  y  t  c  c  q  h  t  d  n  f
c  r  a  k  o  y  u  p  t  j  e  k  r  n
h  p  n  c  o  u  d  o  n  i  b  b  i  m
g  d  g  a  s  t  o  u  f  r  g  c  o  i
e  r  e  p  s  m  r  i  x  j  b  j  e  r
y  n  u  n  s  s  t  c  f  k  c  p  s  i
n  z  s  u  e  o  n  t  x  t  t  w  g  b
i  n  t  e  n  s  i  v  e  e  b  n  a  h
b  u  l  m  l  e  r  r  p  x  m  y  e  e
x  l  u  h  l  v  e  o  m  a  m  s  m  l
k  x  j  n  i  a  r  l  w  j  s  g  d  i
y  l  a  o  v  j  u  u  r  i  p  k  a  z
```

6. Explain the nursing assistant's role in the discharge of a resident

Multiple Choice.
Circle the letter of the correct answer.

1. When does a resident's discharge from the facility become official?
   a. After the doctor writes the discharge order that releases the resident to leave the facility
   b. After the resident is informed of the discharge
   c. After the resident leaves the facility
   d. When the nurse gives the resident instructions to be followed after discharge

2. All of the following are the nursing assistant's responsibility during discharge EXCEPT:
   a. Collecting and packing the resident's belongings
   b. Giving the resident any special dietary instructions
   c. Being positive and reassuring about the change
   d. Moving the resident to his car

3. A nursing assistant is responsible for the resident until:
   a. The discharge order has been written by the doctor.
   b. The resident's items are packed and the inventory list has been checked.
   c. The resident is outside the facility.
   d. The resident is safely in the car with the doors closed.

Short Answer.

1. Explain what it means when a resident leaves a facility AMA.

   _____

   _____

   _____

   _____

   _____

   _____

2. What are three signs that a resident wants to leave the facility?

   _____

   _____

   _____

   _____

   _____

   _____

   _____

   _____

   _____

   _____

   _____

7. Describe the nursing assistant's role during physical exams

Fill in the Blank.
Fill in the correct word in each blank below.

1. Exams can cause _____
   and _____.
   Help residents by _____ to
   them, _____ to
   them, or even holding their hands.

2. A nursing assistant may gather equipment for a physical exam, including a(n)

   _____

   for blood pressure, a(n)

   _____

   (to examine the outer ear and eardrum), and
   a(n) _____

   _____

   (tests for blood in stool).

3. The nursing assistant will place the resident in the correct

   _____

   and stay with the resident as needed.

4. The _____

   _____

   position is used to examine the breasts, chest, abdomen, and perineal area.

5. The nursing assistant will provide

   _____

   measures, such as the privacy screen or

   _____

   and closing the _____.

6. The nursing assistant will hand

   _____

   to the doctor or nurse as needed.

10
Bedmaking and Unit Care

1. Review the key terms in Learning Objective 1 before completing the workbook exercises

2. Discuss the importance of sleep

Fill in the Blank.
Fill in the correct word in each blank below.

1. _____ is a natural period of rest for the mind and body during which _____ is restored.

2. Sleep is needed to replace old _____ with new ones and provide new energy to _____.

3. _____ help the brain sort out all of the things that it has been dealing with during the day.

4. _____ are natural rhythms and cycles related to body functions.

5. The _____ is the 24-hour day-night cycle.

3. Describe types of sleep disorders

Matching.
Write the letter of the correct definition beside each term.

a. Talking during sleep

b. Grinding and clenching the teeth

c. Sleepwalking

d. Inability to fall asleep or to remain asleep

e. Sleep disorders

f. Talking, often along with violent movements, during REM sleep

1. ____ REM sleep behavior disorder

2. ____ Insomnia

3. ____ Sleeptalking

4. ____ Parasomnias

5. ____ Somnambulism

6. ____ Bruxism

4. Identify factors affecting sleep

Scenario.
Read the following scenario and answer the questions that follow.

New resident Anne Ross has been having trouble sleeping. She generally has dinner, dessert, and coffee around 8:30 p.m. every day. Her husband recently died in the home they shared together for 24 years. After his death, she started a new medication to help with her depression. Her roommate, Riva, likes to sleep with the light on because she frequently has to use the bathroom. Sometimes Riva is unable to make it to the bathroom in time and has to call a nursing assistant for assistance. The nursing assistant will change the sheets and help Riva clean herself as quickly as possible.

1. List five factors that could be affecting Anne's ability to sleep.

_____

_____

_____

_____

_____

_____

_____

Name: _____

_____

_____

2. For each factor you listed above, suggest a solution that might help Anne to sleep better.

_____

_____

_____

_____

_____

_____

_____

_____

_____

3. List four problems that can be caused by not sleeping well.

_____

_____

_____

_____

_____

_____

_____

_____

5. Describe a standard resident unit and equipment

Fill in the Blank.
For each of the following, mark an X beside the standard equipment you will see in most resident units.

1. ____ Overbed table

2. ____ Mechanical lift

3. ____ Call light

4. ____ Children

5. ____ Bed

6. ____ Bedpan

7. ____ Massage table

8. ____ Emesis basin

True or False.
Circle the "T" for true or the "F" for false for each of the following statements.

1. T F A nursing assistant must always knock and wait for permission before entering a resident's room.

2. T F Residents' personal items are not very important to them.

3. T F If a safety hazard exists in a resident's room, the nursing assistant should remove it immediately.

4. T F Personal articles must be kept separate from basins, urinals and bedpans in the bedside stand.

5. T F Bedpans should be placed on overbed tables.

6. Explain how to clean a resident unit and equipment

Multiple Choice.
Circle the letter of the correct answer.

1. General care of the resident's unit must be done:
   a. Once a day
   b. Whenever it is needed throughout the day
   c. Once a week
   d. Only when the resident asks

2. All of the following are disposable equipment EXCEPT:
   a. Paper gowns
   b. Cups
   c. Bedpans and urinals
   d. Tissues

3. The call light must always be kept:
   a. Within the resident's reach
   b. Near the door
   c. On the bedside stand
   d. On the overbed table

4. When a resident is transferred, discharged or dies, the nursing assistant is responsible for all of the following EXCEPT:
   a. Repairing damaged or broken furniture
   b. Removing equipment and supplies
   c. Making the bed
   d. Cleaning unit equipment following facility policy

7. Discuss types of beds and demonstrate proper bedmaking

True or False.

1. T F Some beds have built-in scales for weighing bedridden residents.

2. T F Wrinkles, soiled linens, and lumps in beds can cause pressure sores and must be avoided.

3. T F A nursing assistant should wear gloves when removing soiled linens.

4. T F Clean linen should be carried away from a nursing assitant's uniform.

5. T F Linen can be transferred from one resident's room to another resident's room.

6. T F Bed linen should be shaken to clean it of any microorganisms.

7. T F An open bed is made for a resident who will be out of bed all day.

8. T F It is easier to make an occupied bed than an unoccupied bed.

9. T F A nursing assistant should roll dirty linen away from her as it's removed from the bed.

11
Positioning, Moving, and Lifting

1. Review the key terms in Learning Objective 1 before completing the workbook exercises.

2. Explain body alignment and review the principles of body mechanics

Word Search.
Fill in each of the blanks below and find your answers in the word search.

1. _____
   the load.

2. Think ahead, _____
   and communicate the move.

3. Check base of _____
   and be sure to have firm
   _____.

4. _____
   what is being lifted.

5. Keep back _____.

6. Begin in a squatting position and lift with
   the _____.

7. _____
   stomach muscles when beginning the lift.

8. Keep the object _____
   to the body.

9. Do not _____,
   as it increases stress on the back.

10. _____
    or _____
    when possible rather than lifting.

```
s  y  s  s  o  l  r  q  s  o  u  h  z  l
o  t  r  o  p  p  u  s  h  a  u  y  n  c
f  e  r  i  l  d  q  m  f  o  o  l  i  m
a  j  u  a  o  t  w  z  p  k  q  e  d  x
f  n  n  i  i  i  m  f  q  w  f  h  q  d
m  n  a  f  t  g  s  w  f  o  w  f  b  r
j  b  k  s  d  h  h  u  o  q  j  m  n  p
o  t  w  i  s  t  c  t  k  c  z  h  p  j
m  w  u  n  l  e  i  b  e  l  r  t  j  e
q  s  e  s  h  n  s  e  b  g  k  x  i  i
q  j  v  w  g  s  y  s  c  p  u  e  k  v
v  v  d  u  w  e  i  o  b  w  d  e  t  h
r  p  p  r  p  u  l  l  z  l  c  h  y  i
o  e  c  y  t  p  e  c  a  f  a  w  e  z
```

3. Explain why position changes are important for bedbound residents and describe basic body positions

Matching.
Write the letter of the correct definition beside each term.

a. Semi-sitting position in which the head and shoulders are elevated and the resident's knees may be flexed and elevated

b. An extra sheet placed on top of the bottom sheet to help prevent skin damage caused by shearing

c. Helping residents into positions that promote comfort and good health

d. Position in which resident is lying on the abdomen, or front side of the body

e. Position that may be used for a resident who needs a faster emptying of the stomach due to a digestive problem

62

Name: _____

f. Moves the resident into a sitting position on the side of the bed with the legs hanging over the side

g. Position in which a resident is lying on either side

h. Left side-lying position in which the lower arm is behind the back

i. Position in which the resident lies flat on his back

j. Rubbing or friction resulting from the skin moving one way and the bone underneath it remaining fixed or moving in the opposite direction.

k. Position that may be used for a resident who has gone into shock and has poor blood flow

l. Method of turning a resident as a unit while keeping the spine straight

1. _____ Dangling

2. _____ Draw sheet

3. _____ Fowler's

4. _____ Lateral/side

5. _____ Logrolling

6. _____ Positioning

7. _____ Prone

8. _____ Reverse Trendelenburg

9. _____ Shearing

10. _____ Sims'

11. _____ Supine

12. _____ Trendelenburg

Short Answer.
Answer the following questions in the space provided.

1. Why is it important to reposition and turn bedbound residents often?

_____

_____

_____

_____

2. List three things that a nursing assistant should check a resident's skin for each time a resident is repositioned.

_____

_____

_____

_____

_____

_____

_____

4. Describe how to safely transfer residents

Multiple Choice.
Circle the letter of the correct answer.

1. How should a nursing assistant transfer a resident who has a strong side and a weak side?
   a. The weaker side moves first.
   b. The strong side moves first.
   c. It does not matter which side moves first.
   d. A resident with one weak side cannot be transferred.

2. The science of designing equipment and setting up areas to make them safer and to suit the worker's abilities is called:
   a. Transfer
   b. OSHA
   c. Ergonomics
   d. MSD

3. OSHA's ergonomic guidelines include all of the following EXCEPT:
   a. Manual lifting and transferring of residents should be increased as much as possible.
   b. Proper equipment should be available in facilities.
   c. Staff should be trained on equipment and use it as much as possible to avoid injury.
   d. Staff should always have enough help when moving and lifting residents.

4. All of the following are true of transfer belts EXCEPT:
   a. They are called a gait belt when used to help residents walk.
   b. They are used most often for residents with fragile bones or recent fractures.
   c. They fit around the resident's waist, over his clothes.
   d. They give a nursing assistant something firm to hold onto when assisting with transfers.

5. Sliding boards are used for:
   a. Transferring residents who cannot bear weight on their legs from one sitting position to another
   b. Helping residents ambulate
   c. Easier lifting of residents
   d. Transferring residents who have had abdominal surgery

6. All of the following are guidelines for wheelchair use EXCEPT:
   a. A resident's hips should be at the very back of the chair.
   b. When moving down a ramp, go down forward, with the resident facing the bottom of the ramp.
   c. When using an elevator, turn the chair around so that the resident faces forward.
   d. The pocket in the back of the wheelchair can be used to store a resident's chart during transfer.

7. Mechanical lifts are used:
   a. To help protect staff and residents from injury during lifting and moving
   b. To transfer a resident who is severely ill into an ambulance
   c. To transfer a resident onto a stretcher
   d. To transfer a resident into a vehicle

8. For a resident to be able to use a toilet, he must be able to:
   a. Walk to the toilet without assistance
   b. Stand up without assistance
   c. Bear some weight on his legs
   d. Transfer himself from a wheelchair to the toilet without assistance

5. Discuss ambulation

Short Answer.

1. What can a resident who is ambulatory do?

   _____

   _____

   _____

2. List six things that are improved by ambulation and exercise.

   _____

   _____

   _____

   _____

   _____

   _____

3. List three guidelines for helping a visually-impaired resident walk.

   _____

   _____

   _____

   _____

   _____

   _____

   _____

12
Personal Care

1. Review the **key terms** in Learning Objective 1 before completing the workbook exercises

2. Explain personal care of residents

True or False.
Circle the "T" for true or the "F" for false for each of the following statements.

1. T F Good grooming can help keep a person clean and healthy.

2. T F The nursing assistant will make all the decisions about how to groom a resident.

3. T F A resident's preferences regarding bathing must be considered.

4. T F Toileting assistance should be offered during a.m. care but not during p.m. care.

5. T F "Grooming" is the term to describe methods of keeping the body clean, while "hygiene" includes practices like fingernail, foot, and hair care.

6. T F Nursing assistants never help residents with ADLs.

7. T F If a resident takes a long time with personal care tasks, the nursing assistant should do everything for him.

8. T F Residents may be embarrassed by having someone else provide personal care.

9. T F Residents have the right to choose what they want to wear, including jewelry.

10. T F Residents should be left alone during bathing to promote independence.

3. Describe different types of baths and list observations to make about the skin during bathing

Short Answer.
Answer each of the following questions in the space provided.

1. List the four basic types of baths. For each one, list one type of resident for which this bath is suited.

_____
_____
_____
_____
_____
_____
_____
_____

2. How is the decision about which kind of bath a resident will receive made?

_____
_____
_____
_____
_____
_____

3. List ten things to observe and report during personal care and bathing.

_____
_____
_____

Name: _____

_____
_____
_____
_____
_____
_____
_____
_____
_____
_____

4. Explain safety guidelines for bathing

Word Search.

Fill in each of the blanks below and find your answers in the word search.

1. A nursing assistant should not try to

    _____

    a resident alone if he does not believe he can handle the task.

2. Residents should be kept

    _____

    while being transported to the tub or shower room.

3. Make sure the floor in the shower or tub room is _____. Wipe up any _____ or wet areas.

4. Place _____ mats in regular tubs.

5. Check to see that _____ _____ and _____ _____ are secure and in proper working order.

6. Bath _____ and _____ can create slippery surfaces and can put residents at risk of falling.

7. Check water temperature with a

    _____ _____

    or on the wrist.

8. Do not use _____ _____ near a water source.

```
n m e c t s w c b j y t l w
f s l i a r d n a h s f t g
s h e h t a b s t d d y f j
m g c k s b r c h v t s c t
i g t d l b u e t i b t x c
f n r q e a g v h m d q j g
e y i z g r h d e b d a b b
h k c o y g e n r i l p e c
e n a f m v p v m d o g i e
e m l t x d g p o z c a p e
j c a z n f z i m c a j x s
h m p b a o k i e k a d x i
h s p l z l e k t m a r o g
l j l w n e r k e m t y y d
c p i l s n o n r e x p b m
o h a k i m i n r t f k e y
x w n h o p l o q x w f f c
w t c i x n s a z k k c v j
q o e g o r q m x a x f l l
r z s w a p q c e f y b y d
```

5. List the order in which body parts are washed during bathing

Short Answer.

1. Why is it important to follow a specific order when bathing a person?

    _____
    _____
    _____
    _____

2. State the general rule of the order of parts for bathing.

    _____
    _____
    _____
    _____

Labeling.

Look at the figure below. In the blanks provided, number the parts of the body in the order in which they should be bathed.

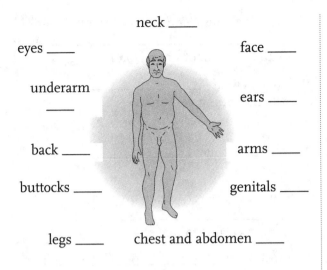

neck _____

eyes _____

face _____

underarm
_____

ears _____

back _____

arms _____

buttocks _____

genitals _____

legs _____   chest and abdomen _____

6. Explain how to assist with bathing

Multiple Choice.
Circle the letter of the correct answer.

1. All of the following are benefits of regular bathing EXCEPT:
    a. Promotes good health and hygiene
    b. Increases circulation
    c. Provides an opportunity to observe the skin
    d. Prevents dryness of skin if done every day

2. All of the following parts of the body should be washed every day EXCEPT:
    a. Hair
    b. Hands
    c. Face
    d. Perineal area

3. When is a partial bath performed?
    a. Every day
    b. Only for testing purposes
    c. On days when a complete bed bath, tub bath, or shower is not done
    d. When a resident cannot get out of bed

4. To shampoo hair for a resident on a stretcher, the nursing assistant should:
    a. Transfer the resident to a bed
    b. Transfer the resident to a chair in front of the sink
    c. Bring the stretcher to the sink and adjust the height of the stretcher
    d. A resident on a stretcher cannot have his hair shampooed

5. What kind of equipment is used to help a resident into a whirlpool bath?
    a. Gait belt
    b. Sliding board
    c. Chairlift
    d. Wheelchair

7. Describe how to perform a back rub

True or False.

1. T F It is inappropriate for a nursing assistant to give a resident a back rub.

2. T F Back rubs help relax muscles and improve circulation.

3. T F Back rubs will be given to all residents.

4. T F All residents will prefer to lie on their stomachs during a back rub.

5. T F Red areas over bony parts of the body should be massaged using long, smooth strokes.

8. Explain guidelines for performing good oral care

Matching.
Write the letter of the correct definition beside each term listed below.

a. Inflammation of the gums

b. Substance that forms on the teeth in a brief period of time

c. Risk of these may be reduced by quality oral care

d. Bad-smelling breath

e. Hard deposits on teeth that are filled with bacteria and may cause gum disease and loose teeth

f. Lacking teeth

1. _____ Edentulous

2. _____ Gingivitis

3. _____ Halitosis

4. _____ Plaque

5. _____ Respiratory infections

6. _____ Tartar

Name: _____

Short Answer.

1. List seven signs and symptoms to report during oral care.

   _____

   _____

   _____

   _____

   _____

   _____

   _____

2. List five ways that a nursing assistant will assist a resident who can brush his own teeth.

   _____

   _____

   _____

   _____

   _____

   _____

   _____

   _____

9. Define "dentures" and explain care guidelines

Crossword Puzzle.
Fill in each of the blanks below and use your answers to complete the crossword puzzle.

Across.

2. Dentures must always be stored in

   _____ _____

   so that they do not dry out and warp.

4. If residents' dentures break, they cannot

   _____.

7. _____ are artificial teeth.

8. After cleaning dentures, store them in a(n)

   _____ _____

   with the resident's name on it.

9. Always wear _____
   when cleaning dentures.

Down.

1. Hot water may _____
   dentures.

3. Dentures are very expensive and

   _____ _____

   for a specialist to make.

5. A(n) _____ is a type of dental appliance that replaces missing or pulled teeth.

6. Dentures may _____
   if left uncovered.

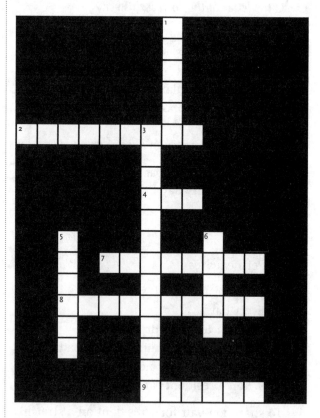

10. Discuss guidelines for performing oral care for an unconscious resident

Multiple Choice.

1. Oral care needs to be done frequently for residents who are unconscious for all of the following reasons EXCEPT:

a. Too much moisture collects in the mouth

b. To remove sordes on the lips, gums, and teeth

c. The mouth becomes dry due to lack of oral fluids, breathing through the mouth, and oxygen therapy

d. To keep the mouth clean and moist

2. Aspiration is:

a. A crust that appears on the lips, gums, and teeth of people who are unconscious

b. A cause of unconsciousness

c. Inhalation of food or drink into the lungs

d. A substance that forms on the teeth

3. One way to prevent aspiration is to:

a. Turn unconscious residents on their backs before beginning oral care

b. Avoid performing oral care on unconscious residents

c. Use as little liquid as possible during oral care

d. Use swabs soaked in large amounts of fluid to clean the mouth

4. A resident who is unconscious may still be able to:

a. Hear

b. Speak

c. Ambulate

d. Feed themselves

5. When providing eye care for an unconscious resident, do all of the following EXCEPT:

a. Use gloves and clean washcloths and towels when bathing the eye.

b. Wipe from the inner aspect to the outer canthus of the eye.

c. Use the same cotton ball to clean both eyes.

d. Follow the care plan and special instructions regarding placing moist compresses on the eyes.

11. Explain how to assist with grooming

True or False.

1. T F Appearance has very little to do with how people feel about themselves.

2. T F The nursing assistant will make all the decisions about how to groom a resident.

3. T F A nursing assistant must always wear gloves when shaving residents.

4. T F Whether a nursing assistant shaves a resident or not depends upon the nursing assistant's preferences.

5. T F Disposable shaving products should be discarded in the biohazard container.

6. T F A disposable razor is the safest and easiest razor to use.

7. T F Fingernails can collect microorganisms or scratch residents, visitors and staff.

8. T F A nursing assistant should cut residents' toenails regularly.

9. T F The application of makeup should be based on residents' wishes.

10. T F Hair care does not affect how residents feel about themselves.

11. T F Nursing assistants should comb residents' hair into childish styles.

12. T F Lice will typically not spread very quickly in a facility.

13. T F If a resident has one side of the body that is weaker than the other, it should be referred to as the "affected" or "involved" side.

14. T F When dressing a resident with one strong side and one weak side, always begin with the strong side.

15. T F Residents will be more comfortable if they wear pajamas all day long.

Name: _____

13
Vital Signs

1. Review the key terms in Learning Objective 1 before completing the workbook exercises

2. Discuss the relationship of vital signs to health and well-being

Matching.
Match each normal range with the appropriate vital sign.

a. 100/60 – 139/89

b. 97.6° F – 99.6° F

c. 60-100 per minute

d. 12-20 per minute

e. 98.6° F – 100.6° F

f. 96.6° – 98.6° F

1. ____ Oral temperature

2. ____ Blood pressure

3. ____ Rectal temperature

4. ____ Pulse rate

5. ____ Respiration rate

6. ____ Axillary temperature

Short Answer.
Answer each of the following questions in the space provided.

1. List the five vital signs.

_____

_____

_____

_____

_____

2. Why is it important to report changes in vital signs to the nurse?

_____

_____

_____

_____

_____

3. Identify factors that affect body temperature

Multiple Choice.
Circle the letter of the correct answer.

1. All of the following are factors that affect body temperature EXCEPT:
    a. Age
    b. Amount of exercise
    c. Environment
    d. Hair color

2. Severe sub-normal body temperature is called:
    a. Circadian rhythm
    b. Hypothalamus
    c. Hypothermia
    d. Fever

3. Signs and symptoms of a fever include all of the following EXCEPT:
    a. Pale skin
    b. Headache
    c. Fatigue
    d. Chills

4. List guidelines for taking body temperature

Fill in the Blank.
Mark an "X" by each person for whom an oral temperature should NOT be taken.

1. ____ Person is confused or disoriented.

Name: _____

2. ____ Person has sores and swelling in his mouth.

3. ____ Person is 40 years old.

4. ____ Person is unconscious.

5. ____ Person has a broken leg.

6. ____ Person is likely to have a seizure.

7. ____ Person has a nasogastric tube.

8. ____ Person has had children.

Fill in the Blank.

For each statement below, write an "O" if it refers to oral temperature, an "R" for rectal temperature, a "T" for tympanic temperature, an "A" for axillary temperature, or "TA" for temporal artery.

1. ____ The most common site for taking temperature

2. ____ Thermometer is usually color-coded red

3. ____ Temperature is registered within seconds

4. ____ Non-invasive method of measuring temperature

5. ____ May be necessary for unconscious residents

6. ____ Thermometer is inserted only ¼ to ½ inch

7. ____ Site for taking temperature is the armpit

8. ____ Considered to be most accurate

9. ____ Ear wax may cause an inaccurate reading

10. ____ Thermometer must be lubricated and inserted no more than one inch

11. ____ Thermometer is usually color-coded green or blue

12. ____ Probe is moved straight across the forehead

13. ____ Considered to be least accurate

14. ____ Site for taking temperature is the ear

15. ____ Ear injury is possible

5. Explain pulse and respirations

Matching.

Write the letter of the correct definition beside each term listed below.

a. The absence of breathing

b. Widen

c. Process that consists of inspiration and expiration

d. Difficulty breathing

e. Inhaling air into the lungs

f. Pulse that is too low

g. Abbreviation for beats per minute

h. Exhaling air out of the lungs

i. Shortness of breath when lying down that is relieved by sitting up

j. Respiration with periods of apnea lasting at least 10 seconds, alternating with periods of slow, irregular breathing and rapid, shallow breathing

k. Pulse that is too high

l. Normal respirations

m. Rapid respirations

1. ____ Apnea

2. ____ BPM

3. ____ Bradycardia

4. ____ Cheyne-Stokes respiration

5. ____ Dilate

6. ____ Dyspnea

7. ____ Eupnea

8. ____ Expiration

9. ____ Inspiration

10. ____ Orthopnea

11. ____ Respiration

12. ____ Tachycardia

13. ____ Tachypnea

6. List guidelines for taking pulse and respirations

Multiple Choice.

1. The most common site for counting pulse beats is:
   a. Apical pulse
   b. Radial pulse
   c. Brachial pulse
   d. Femoral pulse

2. Respiration rate is counted directly after taking the pulse because:
   a. People tend to breathe more quickly if they know they are being observed.
   b. People tend to breathe more slowly if they know they are being observed.
   c. Breathing tends to be more regular if the person knows they are being observed.
   d. It saves time for the nursing assistant.

3. If the radial pulse is less than the apical pulse, this may indicate:
   a. Heart disease
   b. Infection
   c. Fever
   d. Poor circulation to extremities

7. Identify factors that affect blood pressure

Crossword Puzzle.
Fill in each of the blanks below and use your answers to complete the crossword puzzle.

Across.

2. People with _____ have elevated systolic and/or diastolic blood pressure.

5. Blood pressure is the measure of the _____ of the blood against the walls of blood vessels.

6. The bottom number in a blood pressure reading is called the _____ blood pressure.

7. The walls of blood vessels are called _____.

9. The left _____ of the heart causes the blood to surge out of the heart and travel through the body.

10. Regular _____ and being active may decrease blood pressure.

Down.

1. _____ means that a person does not have high blood pressure now but is likely to have it in the future.

3. The top number in a blood pressure reading is called the _____ blood pressure.

4. Being _____ and eating unhealthy diets increase blood pressure.

8. Long-term, chronic _____ appears to raise blood pressure.

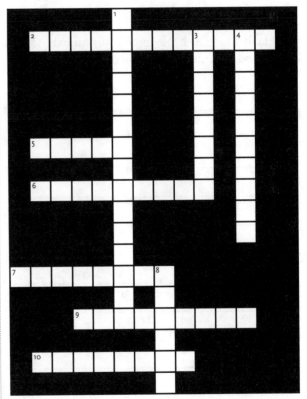

8. List guidelines for taking blood pressure

True or False.
Circle the "T" for true or the "F" for false for each of the following statements.

1. T F   Blood pressure is measured with a device called a sphygmomanometer.

2. T F   The cuff must be the proper size and put on the arm correctly to get an accurate reading.

3. T F An aneroid sphygmomanometer displays readings digitally.

4. T F The apical pulse is used to take a blood pressure reading.

5. T F A blood pressure reading should not be taken on an arm that has a cast or is being used for dialysis.

6. T F If LSS blood pressure readings are ordered for a resident, readings will be taken while he is lying down, sitting, and standing.

9. Describe guidelines for pain management

Short Answer.

1. Have you ever been in pain for an extended period of time? If so, how did it affect your life?

_____

_____

_____

_____

_____

_____

_____

_____

2. Why is pain called the "fifth vital sign?"

_____

_____

_____

_____

_____

3. List five questions that a nursing assistant should ask when helping a resident manage pain.

_____

_____

_____

_____

_____

_____

_____

_____

_____

_____

4. List ten signs that a resident is in pain.

_____

_____

_____

_____

_____

_____

_____

_____

_____

_____

_____

_____

_____

_____

Fill in the Blank.
Looking at measures to reduce pain, fill in each of the following blanks.

1. Offer warm _____
   or _____.

2. Be _____,
   caring, gentle, and _____.

3. Offer _____ _____
   frequently.

4. _____
   the resident's response to pain medication.

5. Assist in frequent changes of
   _____.

6. Report any complaints of _____
   or _____ _____
   promptly to the nurse.

14
Nutrition and Fluid Balance

1. Review the key terms in Learning Objective 1 before completing the workbook exercises

2. Describe common nutritional problems of the elderly and the chronically ill

Crossword Puzzle.
Fill in each of the blanks below and use your answers to complete the crossword puzzle.

Across.

4. Some specific illnesses, such as stroke or multiple _____, make eating and swallowing difficult.

5. Problems with teeth or _____ or poor oral hygiene make chewing difficult.

6. Malnutrition can result from insufficient food intake or an improper _____.

8. Aging and illness affect

    _____,

    or the taking in and using of food by the body to maintain health.

9. _____, or difficulty swallowing, may contribute to a lack of appetite.

Down.

1. A decrease in _____

    _____ and mobility can cause lack of appetite or constipation.

2. _____

    is the lack of proper nutrition.

3. Swallowing problems increase risk of

    _____, or inhalation of food or drink into the lungs.

7. _____ can have side effects for the digestive system.

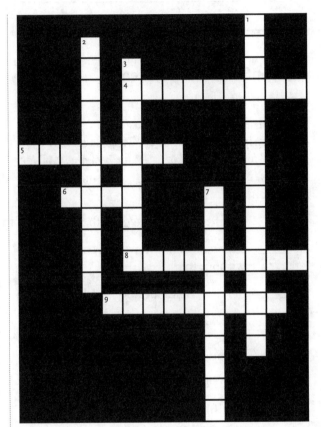

3. Describe cultural factors that influence food preferences

Short Answer.
Answer each of the following questions in the space provided.

1. List four factors that influence food choices.

    _____

    _____

    _____

    _____

    _____

    _____

    _____

    _____

    _____

    _____

Name: _____

2. Of the factors you listed above, which one has the most influence on your personal food choices?

_____

_____

_____

4. Identify six basic nutrients

Matching.
Write the letter of the correct basic nutrient beside each description below. Use a "W" for water, "F" for fats, "C" for carbohydrates, "P" for proteins, "V" for vitamins, or "M" for minerals. Letters may be used more than once.

1. ____ Essential for tissue growth and repair

2. ____ A person can survive only a few days without this

3. ____ Serve as insulation for the body

4. ____ The body does not make most of these nutrients; they can only be obtained through food

5. ____ Gives flavor to foods

6. ____ Add fiber to our diets, which helps with elimination

7. ____ Help keep bones and teeth strong

8. ____ Contain many calories and should be used in small amounts

9. ____ Helps remove waste products from cells

10. ____ Supply the body with vital energy

11. ____ Some of these are fat soluble; some are water soluble

12. ____ Most essential nutrient for life

5. Explain the USDA's MyPyramid

Labeling.
Looking at MyPyramid, fill in the six food groups and one additional element of good health.

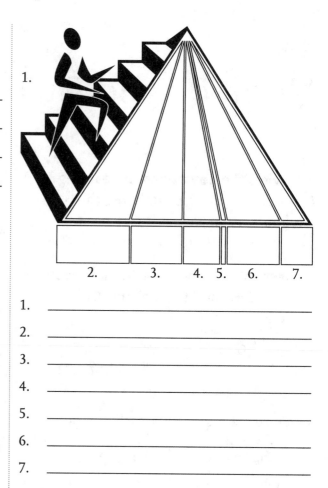

1.

2.   3.   4. 5.   6.   7.

1. _____

2. _____

3. _____

4. _____

5. _____

6. _____

7. _____

Matching.
Read the following descriptions and mark which each is describing – "G" for grains, "V" for vegetables, "F" for fruits, "M" for milk products, "MB" for meat and beans, "O" for oils, or "A" for activity.

1. ____ This group includes foods that retain their calcium content, such as yogurt and cheese.

2. ____ This includes all foods made from wheat, rice, oats, cornmeal, and barley.

3. ____ Foods that are mainly this include mayonnaise, some salad dressings, and soft margarine.

4. ____ One ounce of lean meat or poultry, one egg, or ½ ounce of nuts or seeds can be considered as a one-ounce equivalent from this group.

5. ____ This should be done for at least 30 minutes per day.

6. ____ Important sources of dietary fiber and many nutrients, including folic acid and vitamin C.

7. ____ Most of these eaten should be polyun-saturated (PUFA).

8. ____ At least half of all of these consumed should be "whole."

9. ____ This increases the amount of calories burned.

10. ____ These products are the primary source of calcium, which builds bones and teeth and maintains bone mass.

11. ____ There are five subgroups within this group: dark green, orange, dry beans and peas, starchy, and others.

12. ____ Most choices in this group should be lean or low-fat.

6. Explain the role of the dietary department

Multiple Choice.
Circle the letter of the correct answer.

1. All of the following are responsibilities of the dietary department EXCEPT:
   a. Provide nutritious meals and snacks to residents.
   b. Order special diets for residents.
   c. Prepare food in such a way that residents are able to manage.
   d. Consider residents' likes, dislikes, and nutritional needs.

2. Which of the following information is included on a resident's diet card?
   a. Special diets, allergies, likes and dislikes and other dietary instructions
   b. Intake and output records
   c. Amount of activity
   d. Health department survey results

3. All of the following are guidelines for reading menus to residents and assisting them to fill in their choices EXCEPT:
   a. Speak slowly and clearly.
   b. Answer any questions resident has.
   c. Insist that residents order only nutritious foods.
   d. Make selections sound appetizing.

7. Explain the importance of following diet orders and identify special diets

Short Answer.
For each of the following descriptions, write the kind of diet referred to.

1. Resident is drinking fluids that you can see through.

   _____

2. Resident has kidney or liver disease and is eating vegetables and starches and reducing protein intake.

   _____

3. Resident is eating whole grains and raw fruits and vegetables.

   _____

4. Resident is trying to lose or maintain weight.

   _____

5. Resident is making the transition from a liquid diet to a regular diet.

   _____

6. Resident has severe heart or kidney disease and has fluid intake monitored.

   _____

7. Resident has a serious burn that is healing and is eating meat, fish and cheese.

   _____

8. Resident is taking diuretics and eating bananas, oranges, and sweet potatoes and yams.

   _____

9. Resident has trouble chewing and swallowing and cannot tolerate a regular or soft mechanical diet.

   _____

10. Resident has heart disease and is restricting salt intake.

   _____

11. Resident has a bowel disorder and is decreasing intake of grains, dairy, and coffee.

   _____

12. Resident is consuming clear liquids with the addition of cream soups, milk, and ice cream.

   _____

13. Resident's food is prepared with a blender or food processor.

   _____

14. Resident has intestinal problems and is avoiding spicy foods and citrus fruits.

   _____

15. Resident is trying to gain weight after surgery or an illness.

   _____

16. Resident has heart disease and is eating white meat, skim milk, and low-fat cottage cheese.

   _____

17. Resident has a meal plan that must be followed exactly and must eat everything that is served.

   _____

8. Explain thickened liquids and identify three basic thickening consistencies

True or False.
Circle the "T" for true or the "F" for false for each of the following statements.

1. T F Residents with dysphagia are evaluated to determine if they should consume thickened liquids.

2. T F Thickened liquids move down the throat more slowly and limit the risk of choking.

3. T F Residents who need thickened liquids can drink soda or coffee.

4. T F The three types of thickened liquids generally used by facilities are nectar thick, honey thick, and pudding thick.

5. T F Liquids that are pudding thick can be drunk from a cup with or without a straw.

9. List ways to identify and prevent unintended weight loss

Fill in the Blank.
Fill in the correct word in each blank.

1. Unintended weight loss may be due to a(n) _____ condition or a(n) _____ diet.

2. Unintended weight loss puts a person at a greater risk for _____.

3. It is important to _____ any weight loss you notice.

4. Staff may re-evaluate special _____ orders.

5. Warning signs of unintended weight loss include resident having _____ that do not fit properly or difficulty chewing or _____.

6. Signs that a resident is malnourished include a feeling of _____ throughout the body, frequent _____ and problems with _____.

7. Report any decrease in _____ to nurse.

8. _____ food to the resident's preferences.

10. Describe how to make dining enjoyable for residents

True or False.

1. T F Mealtimes are often the most anticipated times of the day for residents.

2. T F Nursing assistants should encourage residents to eat as little as possible so that they don't gain too much weight.

3. T F Meals do not need to be served at the same time every day.

4. T F Staff should honor residents' requests to sit with friends.

5. T F It does not matter what position residents are in for meals.

6. T F Dining tables should be adjusted to the right height for wheelchairs.

7. T F Food should be served promptly to maintain correct temperature.

8. T F Residents should be given assistive devices for eating if needed.

9. T F If a resident needs his food cut for him before eating, this should be done at the dining table.

10. T F Residents must eat whatever food is served.

11. Describe how to serve meal trays and assist with eating

Multiple Choice.

1. When serving meals to residents, a nursing assistant should:
   a. Check the diet card and identify the resident before serving the meal tray.
   b. Do as much as possible for each resident so that the meal can be finished more quickly.
   c. Leave the door of the food cart open so that the food is not too hot when served.
   d. Serve meals to residents who require the most assistance first.

2. All of the following are ways to promote dignity during mealtimes EXCEPT:
   a. Encourage residents to do whatever they can for themselves.
   b. Provide privacy as needed.
   c. Discourage conversation during mealtimes.
   d. Say positive things about food being served.

3. Guidelines for helping residents during mealtime include:
   a. Insist that residents wear clothing protectors during meals.
   b. Tell the resident which foods look appetizing and which do not.
   c. If food is too hot, blow on it or ask resident to blow on it to cool it.
   d. Respect a resident's refusal to eat.

12. Describe how to assist residents with special needs

Short Answer.
For each of the following problems with eating, list one technique for helping resident to eat.

1. Resident eats too quickly.

   _____

   _____

2. Resident will not stop chewing.

   _____

   _____

3. Resident holds food in his mouth or will not swallow.

   _____

   _____

4. Resident has poor lip closure.

   _____

   _____

5. Resident has no teeth or is missing teeth.

   _____

   _____

6. Resident has dentures that do not fit properly.

   _____

   _____

7. Resident has a change in vision.

   _____

   _____

8. Resident has a protruding tongue or tongue thrust.

   _____

   _____

9. Resident will not open mouth.

   _____

Name: _____

10. Resident falls asleep while eating.

_____

_____

_____

11. Resident chokes when drinking.

_____

_____

_____

12. Resident forgets to eat.

_____

_____

_____

13. Resident drools excessively.

_____

_____

_____

14. Resident tends to lean to one side.

_____

_____

_____

15. Resident tends to fall forward.

_____

_____

_____

13. Discuss dysphagia and list guidelines for preventing aspiration

Multiple Choice.

1. All of the following are causes of dysphagia EXCEPT:
   a. Illness
   b. Medication
   c. Dentures that fit properly
   d. Food choices

2. Signs of dysphagia include all of the following EXCEPT:
   a. Eating very rapidly
   b. Avoidance of eating
   c. Swallowing several times when eating a single bite
   d. Coughing during or after meals

3. Guidelines for preventing aspiration include:
   a. Put residents in a reclining position for eating and drinking.
   b. Place food in the paralyzed side of the mouth.
   c. Offer at least three bites of food before offering a liquid.
   d. Make sure food is swallowed after each bite.

14. Describe intake and output (I&O)

Short Answer.

1. A healthy person generally needs to take in about 64 to 96 oz. of fluid each day. How many mL is this?

2. Ms. Brown just ate some butterscotch pudding from a 6 oz. container. You measure the leftover pudding, which is about 35 mL. How many mL of pudding did Ms. Brown eat?

3. Record this resident's total intake and output:

   1 glass apple juice 140 mL
   1 cup coffee   110 mL
   1 cup soup   170 mL
   Total intake: _____

   11:00 a.m.
   Urinate x 1   220 mL output measured

   1:00 pm
   Urinate x 1   260 mL output measured
   Total output: _____

15. List ways to identify and prevent dehydration

Short Answer.

1. Define dehydration.

_____

_____

_____

_____

2. List ten signs of and symptoms of dehydration.

_____

_____

_____

_____

_____

_____

_____

_____

_____

_____

_____

_____

3. Fill in the POURR acronym for encouraging fluids:

a. P _____

b. O _____

c. U _____

d. R _____

e. R _____

16. List signs and symptoms of fluid overload and describe conditions that may require fluid restrictions

Word Search.

Fill in each of the blanks below and then find your answers in the word search.

1. Fluid overload occurs when more fluid

_____ the body than is _____ from the body.

2. Fluid overload can occur when the heart, _____, or lungs are not working properly.

3. Symptoms of fluid overload include weight _____, difficulty _____, and _____ heart rate.

4. Swelling of the ankles, feet, fingers or hands caused by excess fluid is called _____.

5. _____ is swelling of the abdomen due to excess fluid.

6. Treating fluid overload consists of reduction in _____, a change in the number of _____ the resident sleeps with, and _____ to eliminate the excessive fluid.

7. A(n) _____ _____ order means the person must limit the daily amount of fluids to a level set by the doctor.

8. Reasons for fluid restrictions include recent _____, special _____ _____ ordered, or _____ through a special tube.

```
r u n t c w e x m k x a n k
s e k s b t a q c t b x o y
f b s e t i c s a d m e g k
e b r t d h t c z e m b a s
e q e l r e t b d k r c i j
d e t a n i m i l e g s n l
i r n c v v c a a p x s c f
n o e i x i t t y i y y r c
g i t d n b h g f l l e e o
t y k e q i o j x l f n a q
w n k m n h o t w o u d s n
s u r g e r y f z w y i e l
f n x f f c u w s s r k d c
u f h d l m g e v z r g z s
```

15
The Gastrointestinal System

1. Review the key terms in Learning Objective 1 before completing the workbook exercises

2. Explain key terms related to the body

Matching.
Write the letter of the correct description beside each term listed.

a. Made up of layers of cells; perform specific body functions

b. The study of all life forms

c. Groups of tissues; perform specific functions to keep the body healthy

d. The study of body structure

e. The study of the disorders that occur in the body

f. The condition in which all of the body's systems are balanced and working at their best

g. Basic structural unit of all organisms

h. Made up of different organs that perform specific functions in the body

i. Looks at how body parts function

1. _____ Anatomy

2. _____ Biology

3. _____ Body systems

4. _____ Cells

5. _____ Homeostasis

6. _____ Organs

7. _____ Pathophysiology

8. _____ Physiology

9. _____ Tissues

3. Explain the structure and function of the gastrointestinal system

Word Search.
Fill in the correct answers in the blanks below, then use your answers to complete the word search.

1. The gastrointestinal system is made up of two sections: the

    _____ _____

    and the _____

    _____.

2. Most food and fluids are absorbed in the

    _____ _____.

3. The epiglottis blocks food from entering the
    _____, or _____.

4. Feces is eliminated from the body by
    _____ through
    the _____.

5. The large intestine helps regulate water balance by absorbing _____
    and _____ and
    eliminating solid waste as _____.

6. The functions of the gastrointestinal system are _____ and
    _____ of food,
    _____ of
    nutrients, and
    _____ of waste.

Name: _____

```
u w d c a o c y s r k t t r
h s f c c n q x e d p e c g
m h t l c e v t t r j s a r
i f v o e g a d y k x w r f
p m b n s w o f l x i z t f
d y n o s y n q o j w k l a
g a i i o f c d r s u n a e
s w b t r u e b t x k o n b
d o p s y i e c c b b i i b
g l c e o p n d e r t t t d
l s u g r r q g l s u a s o
v z t i g i p p e u i n e d
j b r d a c s t g s x i t z
f r a n n w n t i o t m n h
d m c f s i a b a o n i i s
x o h v l n n h d l n l o f
m q e l z d i k a k s e r n
o m a x p p q j e o a i t u
i m e f l i c w g b e e s w
s r e u k p h z q h q f a l
s g z j k e w z a z z p g o
```

4. Discuss changes in the gastrointestinal system due to aging

True or False.
Circle the "T" for true or the "F" for false for each of the following statements.

1. T F As a person ages, he may find it harder to taste foods.

2. T F An older person may be constipated more often.

3. T F Difficulty chewing and swallowing may occur as a person ages.

4. T F An increase in the ability to absorb vitamins and minerals is a normal change of aging.

5. T F As a person ages, she may have an increase of saliva and other digestive fluids.

5. List normal qualities of stool and identify signs and symptoms to report about stool

Multiple Choice.
Circle the letter of the correct answer.

1. All of the following are true about bowel movements EXCEPT:
   a. Bowel elimination is the physical process of releasing or emptying the colon or large intestine of stool or feces.
   b. Frequency of bowel movements varies.
   c. It is not important for older people to have regular bowel movements.
   d. Regular bowel movements help prevent serious problems, such as bowel obstructions, from occurring.

2. Normal stool is:
   a. Brown, formed, and tubular in shape
   b. Brown and loose
   c. Reddish and hardened
   d. Tarry and formed

3. All of the following are true of bowel elimination EXCEPT:
   a. There should not be any pain with passing stool.
   b. Residents should not have accidents with passing stool.
   c. A change in the appearance of stool can signal a health problem.
   d. It is normal to see blood or pus in stool.

4. All of the following are signs and symptoms that should be reported to the nurse EXCEPT:
   a. Resident has two bowel movements in one day.
   b. Stool is hard and dry.
   c. Resident has pain with bowel movements.
   d. Resident has fecal incontinence.

6. List factors affecting bowel elimination and describe how to promote normal bowel elimination

Short Answer.

1. List one way each of these factors in this Learning Objective affect bowel elimination: growth and development, psychological factors, diet, fluid intake, physical activity and exercise, personal habits, and medications.

_____

_____

_____

_____

_____

_____

_____

_____

_____

_____

_____

_____

_____

_____

_____

_____

_____

_____

_____

_____

_____

_____

2. What is the difference between a standard bedpan and a fracture pan? How should each be placed?

_____

_____

_____

_____

_____

_____

_____

_____

_____

_____

7. Discuss common disorders of the gastrointestinal system

Matching.
For each of the following descriptions, write the letter of the gastrointestinal disorder referred to.

a. Crohn's disease

b. Constipation

c. Diarrhea

d. Diverticulitis

e. Diverticulosis

f. Fecal/anal incontinence

g. Fecal impaction

h. Flatulence

i. Gastroesophageal reflux disease (GERD)

j. Hemorrhoids

k. Heartburn

l. Irritable bowel syndrome

m. Lactose intolerance

n. Malabsorption

o. Ulcerative colitis

p. Ulcers

1. ____ Causes the wall of the intestines (large or small) to become inflamed

2. ____ Frequent elimination of liquid or semi-liquid feces; BRAT diet is often suggested

3. ____ Occurs when the sphincter muscle which joins the esophagus and the stomach weakens; causes a burning feeling in esophagus directly after meals

4. ____ Inability to digest a type of sugar in milk and other dairy products

5. _____ Enlarged veins in the rectum; symptoms include itching and bleeding during bowel elimination

6. _____ Raw sores in the stomach and small intestine; excessive aspirin use may be a cause

7. _____ Sac-like pouchings of the intestinal wall develop in weakened areas of the wall

8. _____ Chronic condition of the GI tract that is worsened by stress

9. _____ Chronic condition in which the liquid contents of the stomach back up into the esophagus

10. _____ Build-up of dry, hardened feces in the rectum resulting from unrelieved constipation

11. _____ Nutrients from the intestinal tract are not properly absorbed

12. _____ Inability to control the muscles of the bowels, leading to involuntary passage of stool or gas

13. _____ Causes inflammation of and sores in the lining of the large intestine; can cause intestinal bleeding and death if not treated

14. _____ Developed by a small percentage of people with diverticulosis; can cause peritonitis

15. _____ Difficult and often painful elimination of a hard, dry stool

16. _____ Presence of excessive air in the digestive tract

8. Discuss how enemas are given

Fill in the Blank.
Write the correct word in each blank.

1. An enema is given when help is needed _____ _____ from the colon.

2. Enemas are also ordered in preparation for a(n) _____ _____ or _____.

3. _____ water, _____ and _____ enemas are considered cleansing enemas.

4. _____ enemas require more fluid than _____ enemas.

5. Remove the _____ from tubing before inserting it into the rectum.

6. During the enema, the resident should be in the _____ position.

7. Stop immediately if the resident has _____ or if you feel _____.

8. Observe for _____, pain or _____, and the ability to _____ the fluid.

9. The goals of using an oil-retention enema include lubricating the _____, softening _____ for ease of elimination, and reducing _____ with bowel movements.

9. Demonstrate how to collect a stool specimen

True or False.

1. T F A specimen is a sample used for analysis and diagnosis.

2. T F A stool sample may be tested for blood, pathogens, or other things.

3. T F If testing stool for ova and parasites, leave it in the refrigerator overnight before taking it to the lab.

4. T F Specimens may be stored in the same refrigerator as food and drinks.

5. T F Ask the resident not to get urine or toilet paper in the sample.

6. T F A plastic collection container called a "hat" is sometimes inserted into a toilet to collect and measure urine or stool.

7. T F   No special handling is required for collecting a specimen from a resident in isolation.

10. Explain occult blood testing

Fill in the Blank.

1. Hidden or _____ blood is found inside stool with a _____ or a special _____ test.

2. Blood in stool may be a sign of a serious physical problem such as _____.

3. The _____ test checks for occult blood in stool.

4. Specific _____ orders or _____ may be necessary prior to testing.

11. Define the term "ostomy" and identify the difference between colostomy and ileostomy

Short Answer.
Write the correct answer in the space provided.

1. List three reasons an ostomy might be necessary.

_____

_____

_____

_____

_____

2. List three ways to help a person with an ostomy feel better about himself.

_____

_____

_____

_____

_____

_____

_____

12. Explain guidelines for assisting with bowel retraining

Crossword Puzzle.
Fill in the correct answer in each blank, then use your answers to fill in the crossword puzzle.

Across.

2. Take regular trips to the _____ at specific times each day.

6. Keep a record of elimination, including episodes of _____.

8. Most care team members will be involved with _____ and implementing bowel retraining.

9. Be _____ and patient with retraining efforts.

10. Praise attempts and _____ in controlling the bowels.

Down.

1. Never show _____ or anger toward residents who are incontinent.

3. Observe residents' _____ habits.

4. Bowel _____ is the process of assisting residents to regain control of their bowels.

5. Help resident with _____ care as needed.

7. Answer _____ _____ promptly.

9. Provide _____ and do not rush the resident.

Name: _____

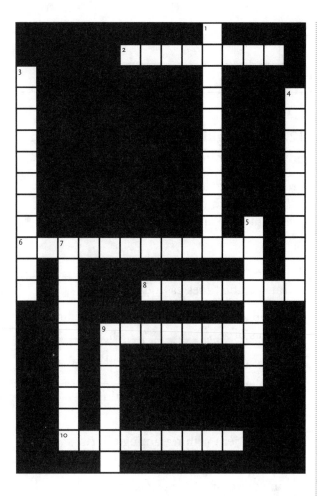

16
The Urinary System

1. Review the key terms in Learning Objective 1 before completing the workbook exercises

2. Explain the structure and function of the urinary system

Fill in the Blank.
Write the correct answers in the blanks below.

1. The kidneys _____ and _____ waste products and _____ materials from the blood.

2. The urinary system consists of two _____, two _____, the urinary bladder and the meatus.

3. Substances not needed by the body, toxins and waste products, stay in the kidney and form _____.

4. The female urethra is _____ than the male urethra.

5. The functions of the urinary system are elimination of _____ products from the blood, maintenance of _____ _____ in the body, regulation of the levels of electroylyes in the body, and assistance in regulation of blood pressure.

3. Discuss changes in the urinary system due to aging

True or False.
Circle the "T" for true or the "F" for false.

1. T F Kidneys not filtering blood as efficiently is a normal change of aging.

2. T F As people age, the bladder holds more urine than it used to.

3. T F Bladder muscle tone weakens with age.

4. T F The bladder may not empty completely as a person ages, increasing the chance of infection.

4. List normal qualities of urine and identify signs and symptoms to report about urine

Multiple Choice.
Circle the letter of the correct answer.

1. All of the following statements are true about urine EXCEPT:
   a. Urine consists of waste products removed from the blood.
   b. Humans need to urinate several times a day to stay healthy.
   c. Urine is normally cloudy when freshly voided.
   d. Urine is normally pale yellow or amber in color.

2. All of the following should be reported to the nurse EXCEPT:
   a. Urine has a faint smell.
   b. Urine is dark or rust-colored.
   c. Resident has pain while urinating.
   d. Resident has episodes of incontinence.

5. List factors affecting urination and describe how to promote normal urination

Short Answer.
List one way each of these factors in this Learning Objective affect bowel elimination: growth and development, psychological factors, fluid intake,

physical activity and exercise, personal habits, medications, and disorders.

_____

_____

_____

_____

_____

_____

_____

_____

_____

_____

_____

_____

_____

_____

_____

_____

_____

_____

_____

_____

_____

6. Discuss common disorders of the urinary system

Matching.
For each of the following descriptions, write the letter of the disorder or treatment referred to.

a. Chronic renal failure (CRF)

b. Dialysis

c. End-stage renal disease (ESRD)

d. Urinary tract infection (UTI)

e. Urine retention

1. ____ Artificial means of removing the body's waste products

2. ____ Inability to adequately or completely empty the bladder

3. ____ A condition in which the kidneys cannot filter waste products from the blood

4. ____ Usually occurs when bacteria enter the urinary tract through the urethra and then begin to multiply in the bladder

5. ____ Occurs when the kidneys have failed and dialysis or transplantation is required

7. Discuss reasons for incontinence

Crossword Puzzle.
Fill in the correct words in the blanks below and use your answers to complete the crossword puzzle.

Across.

4. Because urine is irritating to the skin, _____ residents often.

5. Keep your voice low to keep incontinence a _____ matter.

6. Change wet or _____ clothing immediately.

8. Walking can stimulate the _____ and the need to go to the bathroom.

9. Always refer to incontinence products as _____ or pads.

11. Residents who have incontinence need _____ and understanding.

Down.

1. Follow _____ _____ and the care plan carefully.

2. _____ incontinence is loss of urine due to an increase in intra-abdominal pressure.

3. Nursing assistants must act _____ when handling this problem.

4. Urinary incontinence is the inability to control the muscles of the _____.

7. Incontinence can occur in residents who are confined to bed, ill, or _____.

10. Give good skin care and good _____ care.

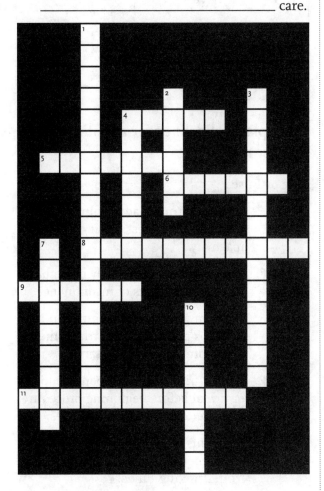

8. Describe catheters and related care

Multiple Choice.

1. A catheter that stays in the bladder for a period of time is called:
   a. Straight catheter
   b. Indwelling catheter
   c. Condom catheter
   d. Texas catheter

2. What is the nursing assistant's role regarding catheters?
   a. Giving daily catheter care
   b. Inserting the catheter
   c. Irrigating the catheter
   d. Removing the catheter

3. All of the following are guidelines for catheter care EXCEPT:
   a. Wear gloves when emptying catheter drainage bags.
   b. Make sure the drainage bag hangs higher then the level of the hips or bladder.
   c. Keep tubing as straight as possible.
   d. Do not try to re-attach a catheter tube that has disconnected.

9. Explain how to collect different types of urine specimens

Matching.
For each of the following descriptions, write the letter of the specimen it refers to. Some letters may be used more than once.

a. Clean-catch urine specimen

b. 24-hour urine specimen

c. Sterile urine specimen

d. Routine urine specimen

1. ____ Collects all urine voided by resident during a 24-hour period

2. ____ First and last urine voided is not included in the sample

3. ____ May be done when a resident has urinary retention

4. ____ Obtained when a resident cannot urinate on his or own

5. ____ Can be collected any time resident voids

6. ____ When beginning test, resident must void and discard first urine

Short Answer.
Write the correct answer in the space provided.

1. How is a specimen collected from a resident with a urostomy?

Name: _____

_____

_____

_____

_____

_____

_____

2. List the five "rights" of specimen collection.

_____

_____

_____

_____

_____

_____

10. Explain types of tests that are performed on urine

Word Search.
Fill in the correct words in the blanks below and find your answers in the word search.

1. A dip strip, also called a _____ strip, tests urine for glucose, pH level, ketones, blood, and specific

    _____.

2. The higher the pH level of a fluid, the more _____ the fluid is.

3. Without _____ to process glucose, _____ build up in the blood and spill into the urine.

4. _____ and
    _____ can
    cause blood to appear in urine.

5. A specific gravity test is done to make sure the _____
    are functioning properly.

6. Urine can be very _____,
    or close to water; it can also be very
    _____, or concentrated.

```
m j q r g z c y h m a b l k
g u k e t o n e s a e s i d
m c x a n r h l w k t j k z
r z p g h i c s p a w r g s
g s s e n l l i n a z d f c
f r y n d m x a j f z p a i
g a e t i y u d k s l r t s
u g n d i l u t e l p k u u
k u d s v v u c p n a k m h
l s i n j j a s o j s j x m
l t k w m z x r n q v e f r
d c l z g w d m g i q n z n
o m w r f q i w c u w n r t
e h l j u m c x u o x w b t
```

11. Explain guidelines for assisting with bladder retraining

True or False.

1. T F Loss of normal bladder function can be caused by illness, injury, or inactivity.

2. T F Residents will not usually be embarrassed by episodes of incontinence.

3. T F Observing residents' elimination habits helps predict when a trip to the bathroom may be necessary.

4. T F Offer a trip to the bathroom, bedpan or urinal before beginning procedures and after completing procedures.

5. T F Residents who have problems with incontinence should be discouraged from drinking fluids.

6. T F Telling a resident how frustrated you are when he is incontinent will encourage him to control his bladder.

7. T F Residents must be encouraged to ask for help with elimination whenever they need it.

17
The Reproductive System

1. Review the key terms in Learning Objective 1 before completing the workbook exercises.

2. Explain the structure and function of the reproductive system

Fill in the Blank.
Write the correct answers in the blanks below.

1. Ova are released from the ovaries each month during the process of

   _____.

2. The male and female reproductive glands are called _____.

3. The female reproductive system produces the female sex cells and the female hormones, _____
   and _____.

4. _____
   is the point at which a woman's menstrual periods stop permanently.

5. The female reproductive system is made up of the _____, fallopian tubes, uterus, _____
   the vulva, and the breasts.

6. The _____
   receives sperm during intercourse and is the outlet for menstrual blood.

7. The male reproductive system consists of the _____, testes, scrotum, epididymis, vas deferens, _____ tissue, seminal vesicle, ejaculatory duct, and _____
   gland.

8. If an ovum is fertilized, it moves into the
   _____, or
   _____.

9. The male reproductive system produces the male hormones, _____
   and _____.

3. Discuss changes in the reproductive system due to aging

True or False.
Circle the "T" for true or the "F" for false.

1. T F A man's prostate gland enlarges with age.

2. T F Menopause is a normal change of aging.

3. T F A woman's production of estrogen and progesterone increases as she ages.

4. T F Number and capability of sperm decrease with age.

5. T F It takes less time for an older man to achieve an erection and to reach orgasm.

6. T F Vaginal walls become drier and thinner; this may cause discomfort during sexual intercourse.

4. Discuss common disorders of the reproductive system

Matching.
Match the letter of the disorder with its symptom(s).

a. Benign prostatic hypertrophy (BPH)

b. Chlamydia

c. Genital herpes

d. Genital HPV infection

e. Gonorrhea

f. Syphilis

g. Trichomoniasis

1. _____ The prostate becomes enlarged and causes feeling of incomplete urination

2. _____ Vaginal discharge and low back pain

3. _____ Symptoms include itching and painful red blisters or open sores

4. _____ Cloudy pus-like discharge from the penis and swelling of the testes

5. _____ Genital warts may appear

6. _____ Small, painless sore on the penis soon after infection

7. _____ Green-yellow vaginal discharge with a strong odor

5. Describe sexual needs of the elderly

Short Answer.
Write the correct answer in the space provided.

1. What is the appropriate attitude for a nursing assistant to have regarding residents' sexual behaviors?

_____

_____

_____

_____

_____

_____

_____

_____

2. What should a nursing assistant do if she encounters a sexual situation?

_____

_____

_____

_____

_____

6. Describe vaginal irrigation.

Word Search
Write the correct answers in the blanks below and find your answers in the word search.

1. Vaginal irrigation, or a vaginal

_____, is a rinsing of the vagina to cleanse the vaginal tract.

2. It is performed prior to

_____ _____

or examinations or due to vaginal

_____.

3. May also introduce _____ into the vagina to treat disorders or reduce

_____.

4. Always provide plenty of _____ for this procedure.

5. Place the resident in the

_____ _____ position.

6. Hold the container not more than

_____ inches over the perineal area.

7. Report pain or discomfort or

_____ swelling to the nurse.

```
v  p  v  a  s  b  f  b  p  v  y  b  s  b
g  s  r  r  l  d  s  d  o  p  j  g  e  g
t  i  g  s  y  f  r  r  x  g  z  p  r  w
t  j  w  l  t  u  e  r  e  l  x  r  u  w
d  r  l  t  n  b  q  q  d  h  e  l  d  a
w  s  o  a  e  y  j  n  z  j  c  l  e  n
l  u  c  f  b  b  n  o  t  l  e  u  c  h
n  t  e  q  m  e  d  i  c  a  t  i  o  n
l  y  r  x  u  o  e  g  a  n  i  a  r  d
l  v  r  e  c  y  c  a  v  i  r  p  p  y
o  y  h  j  e  o  e  s  p  m  t  u  l  b
d  h  z  f  r  v  m  f  i  o  v  f  a  i
j  n  t  x  l  e  r  u  u  d  z  c  c  i
b  p  d  e  a  w  s  d  g  b  q  h  i  c
r  l  w  r  s  t  o  o  j  a  q  b  g  x
x  t  k  a  r  q  i  x  q  p  d  o  r  o
n  p  v  b  o  c  v  g  p  n  u  f  u  p
a  v  n  m  d  b  b  z  v  h  s  a  s  a
```

18
The Integumentary System

1. Review the key terms in Learning Objective 1 before completing the workbook exercises

2. Explain the structure and function of the integumentary system

Fill in the Blank.
Write the correct answers in the blanks below.

1. The skin is the largest _____ in the human body.

2. The substance that gives skin its color is _____.

3. The skin covers and _____ the body, provides _____ through nerves, regulates body temperature, and prevents the loss of too much _____.

4. The two basic layers of the skin are the _____ and _____.

5. _____ are found in the skin that give us the ability to feel and _____.

Short Answer.
Write the correct answer in the space provided.

1. List the parts of the integumentary system.

_____

_____

_____

_____

_____

_____

_____

2. List five functions of the integumentary system.

_____

_____

_____

_____

_____

_____

_____

_____

_____

_____

_____

3. Discuss changes in the integumentary system due to aging

True or False.
Circle the "T" for true or the "F" for false.

1. T F Skin cancer is a normal change of aging.

2. T F The amount of fat and collagen increases with age.

3. T F Skin loses elasticity with age, causing wrinkles.

4. T F Skin becoming thinner and more fragile is a normal change of aging.

5. T F Hair and nail growth slows as people age.

6. T F Brown spots may appear on the skin in areas exposed to the sun.

7. T F Hair thinning and turning gray is not a normal change of aging.

4. Discuss common disorders of the integumentary system

Matching.
For each of the following descriptions, write the letter of the disorder or treatment referred to.

a. Burns

b. Eczema

c. Fungal infections

d. Gangrene

e. Psoriasis

f. Ringworm

g. Scabies

h. Shingles

i. Warts

j. Wounds

1. _____ Caused by tiny mites that burrow into the skin to lay eggs

2. _____ Symptoms include discoloration of the skin, sores that do not heal, loss of feeling, and foul-smelling discharge

3. _____ Rough, hard bumps caused by a virus that invades the skin, usually through a cut or tear

4. _____ Chronic skin condition in which cells of the skin grow too fast, causing red, white, or silver patches to form

5. _____ Usually caused by perspiration

6. _____ There are varying degrees of skin damage; can cause a resident's condition to deteriorate quickly

7. _____ Caused by the same virus that causes chicken pox

8. _____ Topical steroid creams and soothing or drying lotions may be prescribed

9. _____ Fungal infection that causes red scaly patches to appear in a ring shape

10. _____ Types of these include abrasions, avulsions, incisions, lacerations, punctures and contusions

5. Discuss pressure sores and identify guidelines for preventing pressure sores

Word Search.
Fill in the correct answers in the blanks below and find your answers in the word search.

1. Skin breakdown usually occurs at _____ points.

2. Areas of the body where the bone lies close to the skin are called _____ _____.

3. _____ is the death of living cells or tissues caused by lack of nourishment to tissues.

4. Moisture and _____ contribute to skin breakdown.

5. The sores or wounds that result from skin deterioration and shearing are called _____ _____.

6. The first signs of skin breakdown include pale, white, or _____ skin.

7. Pressure sores are much easier to _____ than to cure.

8. Darker skin may look

_____

when skin breakdown begins to occur..

9. _____
linens, as well as crumbs or other irritating objects in the bed increase the risk of pressure sores.

10. Keep skin clean and _____.

11. Assist immobile residents to change position at least every _____ hours.

12. Perform _____ _____ _____ exercises as ordered.

13. Use _____ to separate skin surfaces.

```
l j t i s v b r v o g p q m
v g v n a n o i t c e f n i
i p h o v a n g e p t e l f
g n q i a i y f i s c c e p
u u a t l w p d i p t d r b
w l x o h o r s b c q e k n
x z o m a t o i w v s z d p
n m a f w r m b n s w d t e
w z d o c o i r u k o x o o
g q e e f o n r a q l n l e
x q n g o s e z u w l e m r
b b e n d s n k w a i i d t
j z d a o j c e u w p e j e
u g d r t n e v e r p r c c
o q e x y s s v p b h c x x
a s r p q i c n q d h m t i
```

6. Explain the benefits of warm and cold applications

True or False.

1. T F Hot or cold applications can be either moist or dry.

2. T F The body responds to both heat and cold in the same way.

3. T F Hot applications close blood vessels and cold applications open them.

4. T F You should always wear gloves when assisting with a sitz bath.

5. T F Moist applications are less likely to cause injury than dry applications.

6. T F Residents with high temperatures may need to have a cooling or tepid sponge bath.

7. T F Warm and cold applications should not be applied for more than 20 minutes.

Multiple Choice.
Circle the letter of the correct answer.

1. The benefits of heat include:
   a. It reduces pain and swelling.
   b. It decreases blood flow to the area.
   c. It helps stop bleeding.
   d. It constricts blood vessels.

2. The benefits of cold applications include:
   a. Chills and shivering
   b. It increases blood flow to the area.
   c. It brings down high temperature.
   d. It makes skin cyanotic.

3. How does moisture affect warm and cold applications?
   a. It strengthens the effect.
   b. It weakens the effect.
   c. It has no effect.
   d. It allows use of warm and cold applications for longer than 20 minutes.

4. All of the following are signs that an application is causing tissue damage EXCEPT:
   a. Excessive redness
   b. Blisters
   c. Constriction of vessels
   d. Numbness

7. Discuss non-sterile and sterile dressings

Short Answer.

1. How do open wounds increase the risk of infection?

   _____

   _____

   _____

   _____

   _____

2. List three types of supplies that are considered sterile.

   _____

   _____

   _____

   _____

   _____

   _____

   _____

3. What happens if any part of a sterile field
   becomes contaminated?

_____

_____

_____

_____

_____

_____

_____

_____

Name: _____

19
The Circulatory or Cardiovascular System

1. Review the key terms in Learning Objective 1 before completing the workbook exercises

2. Explain the structure and function of the circulatory system

Word Search.
Write the correct answers in the blanks below and find your answers in the word search.

1. The heart is composed of _____ main chambers: the _____ and the _____.

2. Carbon dioxide is removed in the _____ when we exhale, and _____ is added when we inhale.

3. Blood is made up of solids and liquids: _____ and _____.

4. Blood is pumped from the right _____ to the right ventricle.

5. Platelets cause the blood to _____, preventing excess _____.

6. The function of the heart is to _____ _____ through the blood vessels to every cell.

7. Blood transports _____, _____, and hormones to cells.

8. Plasma is made up of mostly _____.

9. The largest artery in the body is the _____.

10. Blood is composed of three different types of blood cells: red blood cells or _____, white

blood cells or _____, and platelets or _____.

11. _____ gives blood its red color.

```
c c f l j f m f s k l w z g
y a t r o a w s k d m t n a
k j a s b x j i e w u i b g
a i k n r j y q c f d g i x
s c u a f x j g t e o r d h
c e a f v v p r e h o p d f
h l t r q r j l m n l o h v
m l r y n f b m a n b b d e
v s i d c o s b v s p k l n
h f a w t o l c s d m e i t
w a n x z d b u e k u a p r
i m h a d n f m n k p w d i
k r u o f m s z o g c x f c
m u f i g u s c m r s e o l
q e a k r w y e r d h w g e
b w e r y t h r o c y t e s
z k k r e t a w h q k d j l
g a m s d x w w m i m b g i
```

3. Discuss changes in the circulatory system due to aging

True or False.
Circle the "T" for true or the "F" for false.

1. T F   Heart disease is a normal part of aging.

2. T F   The heart pumping less efficiently is a normal part of aging.

3. T F   Blood vessels widen and become more efficient with age.

4. T F   Blood vessels become less elastic as a person ages.

5. T F   As a person gets older, blood flow increases.

Name: _____

4. Discuss common disorders of the circulatory system

Matching.
For each of the following descriptions, write the letter of the disorder or treatment referred to.

a. Anemia

b. Angina pectoris

c. Anti-embolic stockings

d. Congestive heart failure (CHF)

e. Coronary artery disease (CAD)

f. Hypertension (HTN)

g. Ischemia

h. Myocardial infarction (heart attack)

i. Myocardial ischemia

j. Occlusion

k. Orthopnea

l. Peripheral arterial disease (PAD)

m. Peripheral vascular disease (PVD)

n. Prehypertension

o. Pulmonary edema

p. Stable angina

q. Unstable angina (USA)

1. ____ Occurs when the coronary arteries narrow, causing reduced blood supply to the heart

2. ____ Condition in which the red blood cells or hemoglobin in red blood cells is very low

3. ____ Condition in which the heart muscle does not get enough blood and therefore lacks oxygen

4. ____ Prevent swelling and blood clots; increase blood circulation

5. ____ Obstruction of a blood vessel

6. ____ All or part of the blood flow to the heart muscle is blocked, causing muscle cells to die

7. ____ Life-threatening complication of CHF or MI in which fluid builds up in the lungs

8. ____ Most common type of PVD; blockage is caused by buildup of fatty deposits in arterial walls

9. ____ Chest pain or discomfort due to CAD

10. ____ Lack of blood supply to an area

11. ____ Condition in which blood supply to the legs, feet, arms or hands is decreased due to poor circulation

12. ____ Shortness of breath when lying down that is relieved by sitting up

13. ____ Occurs when normal cardiac output cannot meet the needs from ADLs

14. ____ Chest pain that occurs when person is active or under severe stress

15. ____ Chest pain that occurs when a person is at rest and not exerting himself

16. ____ Person does not have high blood pressure now but is likely to in the future

17. ____ When blood pressure consistently measures 140/90 or higher

20
The Respiratory System

1. Review the key terms in Learning Objective 1 before completing the workbook exercises

2. Explain the structure and function of the respiratory system

Fill in the Blank.
Write the correct answers in the blanks below.

1. Two functions of the respiratory system are to _____ oxygen to cells and _____ carbon dioxide from the cells.

2. _____ is the process that consists of inspiration (breathing in) and expiration (breathing out).

3. The epiglottis blocks food from entering the windpipe, or _____.

4. The _____ contract and expand the chest cavity during _____ _____, when we breathe in.

5. The larynx enables humans to _____.

6. The lungs are covered by a membrane called the _____.

7. The exchange of _____ and _____ _____ gases occur in the lungs and in the cells.

8. The process of breathing air in and out is _____; it never stops.

9. The air sacs of the lungs are called the _____.

Short Answer.
Write the correct answer in the space provided.

1. List the parts of the respiratory system.

_____

_____

_____

_____

_____

_____

_____

_____

2. List the four functions of the respiratory system.

_____

_____

_____

_____

_____

_____

_____

3. Discuss changes in the respiratory system due to aging

True or False.
Circle the "T" for true or the "F" for false.

1. T F A decrease in lung capacity is a normal change of aging.

2. T F Asthma is a normal part of aging.

3. T F As a person ages, the air sacs in the lungs become less elastic and decrease in number.

4. T F Airways become more elastic with age, increasing movement of air inside of the lungs.

5. T F When a person gets older his rib cage changes and the chest muscles become weaker.

6. T F With age the cough reflex becomes more effective and cough becomes stronger.

7. T F Oxygen in blood decreases with age.

8. T F A person's voice becomes weaker as she gets older.

4. Discuss common disorders of the respiratory system

Matching.
For each of the following descriptions, write the letter of the disorder or treatment referred to.

a. Acute bronchitis

b. Asthma

c. Bronchiectasis

d. Chronic bronchitis

e. Chronic obstructive pulmonary disease (COPD)

f. Emphysema

g. Multidrug-resistant TB (MDR-TB)

h. Pneumonia

i. Tuberculosis (TB)

1. _____ Caused by an infection and usually treated with antibiotics

2. _____ Highly contagious lung disease that can cause death if left untreated

3. _____ Chronic, progressive disease leading to difficulty breathing due to obstruction of the airways

4. _____ Chronic, episodic disorder with unknown cause; residents may need an inhaler with them at all times

5. _____ Chronic condition that usually results from cigarette smoking and chronic bronchitis

6. _____ Can develop when a person with TB fails to take all of the prescribed medication

7. _____ Serious illness that can result in chronic coughing, shortness of breath, weight loss and coughing up blood

8. _____ Lining of bronchial tubes becomes inflamed, causing scarring of the lining of the bronchial tubes

9. _____ Inflammation of the lungs caused by viral, bacterial, or fungal infection and/or chemical irritants

5. Describe oxygen delivery

True or False.

1. T F Nursing assistants may remove a resident's oxygen if the resident finds it annoying.

2. T F It is safe to smoke around oxygen.

3. T F Oxygen therapy is the administration of oxygen given to increase the supply of oxygen to the lungs.

4. T F Oxygen can be applied or adjusted by nursing assistants.

5. T F Common types of oxygen delivery devices include the nasal cannula, simple face mask, and the oxygen concentrator.

6. T F It is important to perform frequent skin care on areas of the face where oxygen device rests.

7. T F Petroleum-based lubricants are best for soothing sensitive areas on the nose and mouth.

8. T F A nursing assistant should encourage activity as permitted for residents who are receiving oxygen.

9. T F Notify the nurse of sores on the nasal area, complaints of discomfort or pain, and chest pain or tightness.

10. T F All residents using oxygen will need oxygen continuously.

6. Describe how to collect a sputum specimen

Crossword Puzzle.
Fill in the correct answer in the blanks below and enter your answers into the crossword puzzle.

Across.

2. Resident should not rinse with

   _____

   before a sputum specimen collection.

4. _____ _____

   is the best time to collect sputum.

5. Resident should rinse mouth with

   _____

   before obtaining sputum specimen.

6. Sputum is not the same as

   _____,

   which comes from the salivary glands inside the mouth.

Down.

1. Sputum may show evidence of cancer or

   _____.

3. The lab will look for _____
   cells, microorganisms, or blood.

6. A _____ specimen
   comes from inside the respiratory system.

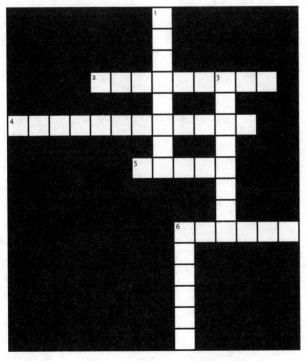

7. Describe the benefits of deep breathing exercises

Short Answer.

1. Why might residents need to do deep breathing exercises?

   _____

   _____

   _____

   _____

   _____

   _____

2. List two possible benefits of regular use of the incentive spirometer.

   _____

   _____

   _____

   _____

   _____

   _____

   _____

   _____

Name: _____

21
The Musculoskeletal System

1. Review the key terms in Learning Objective 1 before completing the workbook exercises

2. Explain the structure and function of the musculoskeletal system

Fill in the Blank.
Fill in the correct answer in each blank below.

1. The musculoskeletal system gives the body _____ and _____.

2. The musculoskeletal system allows the body to _____ and _____ itself, provides _____ for the body and creates _____.

3. Muscles are groups of _____ that help the body move by _____ and _____.

4. _____ are the rigid connective tissues that make up the _____, which is the framework of the human body.

5. _____ are found at the place where two bones come together; they hold bones together and provide _____ and _____.

6. _____ are strong, fibrous bands that connect bones and help _____ the joints and joint _____.

Short Answer.
Answer each of the following questions in the space provided.

1. List the five parts of the musculoskeletal system.

_____
_____
_____
_____
_____
_____
_____

2. List the three types of muscles in the body.

_____
_____
_____
_____
_____
_____
_____
_____
_____
_____

3. List the four types of bones.

_____
_____
_____
_____
_____
_____
_____
_____
_____

Name: _____

4. List the seven functions of the musculoskeletal system.

_____

_____

_____

_____

_____

_____

_____

_____

_____

_____

_____

3. Discuss changes in the musculoskeletal system due to aging

True or False.
Circle either the "T" for true or the "F" for false for each statement below.

1. T F As people age, the body loses muscle mass.

2. T F As people age, bones gain calcium.

3. T F Bones are more easily broken as people age.

4. T F Joints become more flexible with age.

5. T F As people age, height is gradually lost.

4. Discuss common disorders of the musculoskeletal system

Matching.
Match each term below with its correct definition.

a. Amputations

b. Arthritis

c. Bursitis

d. Contracture

e. Flexion

f. Fracture

g. Muscular dystrophy

h. Osteoarthritis

i. Osteoporosis

j. Phantom limb pain

k. Phantom sensation

l. Prosthesis

m. Rheumatoid arthritis

n. Total hip replacement

o. Total knee replacement

p. Traction

1. ____ Condition in which bones lose mass, causing them to be brittle and easily broken

2. ____ Surgical removal of an extremity

3. ____ May be necessary due to damage from injuries or arthritis or to help stabilize a knee that buckles repeatedly

4. ____ An artificial body part that is specially fitted to replace a missing limb or extremity

5. ____ Surgery that replaces the head of the long bone of the leg where it joins the hip

6. ____ General term for the inflammation of the joints that can cause pain, stiffening and swelling

7. ____ Condition in which the small sacs of fluid around the joints become inflamed

8. ____ Hereditary, progressive disease that causes muscles to waste away, decrease in size and weaken

9. ____ Condition that affects the synovial membrane and causes stiffness, swelling, severe pain and deformities which can be severe and disabling

10. ____ Person feels pain in a limb or extremity that has been amputated

11. ____ Bending a body part

12. ____ Permanent and painful stiffening of a muscle

13. ____ Person who has had an amputation may feel itching and tingling in the area where a limb once was

14. ____ Condition in which the cushiony cartilage that rests between the bones and pads the ends of the bones begins to slowly erode

15. ____ A broken bone

16. ____ Method of treating fractures that keeps bones in place

Short Answer.

1. List eight guidelines for preventing falls.

_____

_____

_____

_____

_____

_____

_____

_____

_____

_____

_____

_____

_____

_____

_____

2. List five guidelines for cast care.

_____

_____

_____

_____

_____

_____

_____

_____

_____

_____

3. List six guidelines for care of resident with total hip replacement.

_____

_____

_____

_____

_____

_____

_____

_____

_____

_____

4. Define "partial weight bearing," "non-weight bearing," and "full-weight bearing."

_____

_____

_____

_____

_____

Name: _____

5. Describe elastic bandages

Word Search.
Fill in the correct words in the blanks below and find your answers in the word search.

1. Elastic bandages are also called non -
   _____ or
   self-_____ bandages.

2. Elastic bandages are used to keep
   _____ and
   _____ in place
   and provide _____,
   _____ and support
   for body parts.

3. These bandages are used to decrease
   _____ from
   injuries and keep _____
   bags in place.

4. Elastic bandages must be wrapped snugly
   enough to provide the proper amount of
   compression and _____
   but not so snugly that they interfere with
   _____.

5. Signs and symptoms of poor circulation
   include skin that is _____
   to the touch and _____
   marks on the skin.

```
s u d c i r c u l a t i o n
u p w x n e v v g q g c o e
p i l f d k l e n a j i k b
p a q i e x t i i d s r u h
o g k n n c e c r s k m m n
r n l q t t q e e e o w v t
t i n m a x s r h b t d f a
d l y u t s p l d e h s n g
b l w o i m c c a b f v f b
l e o n o i t c e t o r p m
i w g c n q c u d j s z p z
g s j v m e n r e v n w f d
t c f j h t k m p n n f e n
o c t k i a q c k n f h i g
```

Short Answer.
Fill in the correct words of the "RICE" acronym for reducing pain and swelling when an injury has occurred.

R _____

I _____

C _____

E _____

22
The Nervous System

1. Review the key terms in Learning Objective 1 before completing the workbook exercises

2. Explain the structure and function of the nervous system

Fill in the Blank.
Write the correct answers in the blanks below.

1. The nervous system _____ and _____ all body functions.

2. The nervous system also _____ and _____ information from outside the body.

3. The _____ is the basic working unit of the nervous system.

4. The two main parts of the nervous system are the _____ nervous system and the _____ nervous system.

5. The right side of the brain, or right _____ controls the motor activity on the _____ side of the body, while the left side of the brain, or left _____ controls the motor activity on the _____ side of the body.

6. The peripheral nervous system consists of the _____ and _____ nerves.

7. The _____ and _____ make up the central nervous system.

8. The ear provides _____ and _____.

9. Two functions of the nervous system are that it controls and coordinates mental _____ and provides _____ centers of heartbeat and respiration.

10. The sense organs are part of the nervous system. They include the _____, tongue, _____, eyes and _____.

11. Inside the back of the eye is the _____, which contains cells that respond to light and send messages to the brain.

3. Discuss changes in the nervous system due to aging

True or False.
Circle the "T" for true or the "F" for false.

1. T F Weakened vision is a normal part of aging.

2. T F Some short-term memory loss may occur with age.

3. T F As people age, the senses become stronger.

4. T F Responses and reflexes speed up with age.

5. T F Sensitivity of nerve endings decreases with age, resulting in weakened sense of touch.

6. T F Slight hearing loss is not a normal change of aging.

4. Discuss common disorders of the nervous system

Matching.
For each of the following descriptions, write the letter of the disorder or condition referred to.

a. Age-related macular degeneration

Name: _____

b. Aphasia

c. Cataract

d. Cerebrovascular accident (CVA)

e. Concussion

f. Confusion

g. Delirium

h. Dysphagia

i. Emotional lability

j. Epilepsy

k. Glaucoma

l. Hemiparesis

m. Hemiplegia

n. Hyperopia

o. Multiple sclerosis

p. Myopia

q. One-sided neglect

r. Paraplegia

s. Parkinson's disease

t. Quadriplegia

u. Seizures

v. Transient ischemic attack (TIA)

1. ____ Paralysis on one side of the body

2. ____ Loss of function of the lower body and legs

3. ____ A sudden state of severe confusion due to a change in the body

4. ____ A general term used to describe a pattern of repeated seizures

5. ____ May be caused by tumors, head injuries, or injuries to the brain during birth

6. ____ Difficulty swallowing

7. ____ Temporary or permanent state in which a person is unable to think clearly and logically

8. ____ Condition that causes the area of the eye that allows people to see detail to degenerate

9. ____ The pressure inside the eye increases, causing damage to the optic nerve

10. ____ Develops when the lens of the eye becomes cloudy

11. ____ Ability to see objects that are near more clearly than distant objects

12. ____ Disorder that causes loss of protective covering that protects nerves and spinal cord

13. ____ Caused by obstruction or rupture of a blood vessel cutting off blood supply to the brain

14. ____ Inability to speak or speak clearly

15. ____ Tendency to ignore a weak or paralyzed side of the body

16. ____ Warning sign of CVA

17. ____ Head injury that occurs from a banging movement of the brain against the cranium

18. ____ Progressive disorder that can cause tremors and a mask-like facial expression

19. ____ Inappropriate or unprovoked emotional responses

20. ____ Loss of function of the arms, trunk, and legs

21. ____ Weakness on one side of the body

22. ____ Ability to see distant objects more clearly than objects that are near

True or False.

1. T F Strokes that occur on the right side of the brain affect functioning on the right side of the body.

2. T F Diminished awareness or one-sided paralysis cause a lack of sensation that increases the risk of injury.

3. T F Residents with Parkinson's disease may do range of motion exercises to prevent contractures and strengthen muscles.

4. T F Multiple sclerosis generally occurs in young adulthood.

5. T F Spinal cord injuries are treated with more success if the cord is completely cut or severed.

6. T F A cause for seizure disorders can always be determined.

7. T F It is usually not necessary to treat glaucoma.

5. Discuss dementia and related terms

Multiple Choice.
Circle the letter of the correct answer.

1. Dementia is:
   a. The ability to think clearly and logically
   b. A normal change of aging in the brain
   c. A serious loss of mental abilities that interferes with normal functioning
   d. An increase in cognitive ability

2. The most common form of dementia is:
   a. Parkinson's disease
   b. AIDS
   c. Alzheimer's disease
   d. Excessive alcohol or drug use

3. All of the following statements are true of dementia EXCEPT:
   a. Dementia is always irreversible.
   b. Dementia may affect a person's social skills.
   c. Diagnosing the cause of dementia is difficult.
   d. People who have dementia may develop delirium.

6. Discuss Alzheimer's disease and identify its stages

Short Answer.
Write the correct answer in the space provided.

1. Define Alzheimer's disease and briefly describe how it occurs.

_____

_____

_____

_____

_____

_____

_____

2. List five things that occur in each of the three stages of Alzheimer's disease.

Stage 1: _____

_____

_____

_____

_____

_____

Stage 2: _____

_____

_____

_____

_____

_____

Stage 3: _____

_____

_____

_____

_____

_____

3. Why is it important to encourage independence in residents with Alzheimer's disease?

_____

_____

_____

_____

_____

_____

_____

Name: _____

7. List strategies for better communication with residents with Alzheimer's disease

Crossword Puzzle.
Fill in the correct word in each blank below and use your answers to complete the crossword puzzle.

Across.

2. Watch for _____ cues as the ability to talk lessens.

4. Try to limit the times you say
   " _____."

6. If resident is paranoid or accusing, do not take it _____.

7. If the resident is frightened or anxious, speak in a quiet area with few
   _____.

10. Talk about only one
    _____ at a time.

11. _____ directions and answers as needed.

Down.

1. Repeating words, phrases, questions or actions is called _____.

3. Check your _____
   _____ to
   make sure you are not tense or hurried.

5. Never _____ a resident with Alzheimer's before identifying yourself and greeting him by name.

7. If resident is verbally abusive, remember that it is the _____
   speaking and not the resident.

8. Encourage the resident to point,
   _____, or
   act out what she is trying to say.

9. Using a _____
   tone of voice than normal can be calming.

10. Break tasks into simpler
    _____.

12. Assume that residents with AD are
    _____ of
    the losses in their abilities.

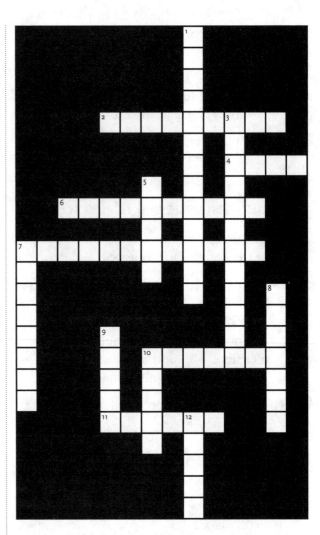

8. Identify personal attitudes helpful in caring for residents with Alzheimer's disease

Short Answer.
For each of the helpful attitudes listed, write one reason why it is important.

1. Do not take it personally.

_____

_____

_____

_____

_____

_____

_____

_____

Name: _____

2. Put yourself in their shoes.

_____
_____
_____
_____
_____
_____
_____
_____
_____

3. Work with the symptoms and behaviors you see.

_____
_____
_____
_____
_____
_____
_____
_____

4. Work as a team.

_____
_____
_____
_____
_____
_____
_____
_____

5. Take care of yourself.

_____
_____
_____
_____
_____
_____
_____

6. Work with family members.

_____
_____
_____
_____
_____
_____
_____
_____

7. Remember the goals of the care plan.

_____
_____
_____
_____
_____
_____
_____
_____

9. Describe guidelines for problems with common activities of daily living (ADLs)

Fill in the Blank.
For each of the following statements, write a "G" if it is a good idea to do this with a resident with Alzheimer's disease or write "B" if it is a bad idea.

1. _____ Use non-slip mats, tub seats, and handholds to ensure safety during bathing.

2. _____ Always bathe the resident at the same time every day, even if he is agitated.

3. _____ Calmly explain what you are doing the same way every time.

4. _____ Do not attempt to groom the resident because she will not understand it.

5. _____ If the resident is incontinent, do not give him fluids.

6. _____ Check the resident's skin regularly for signs of irritation.

7. _____ Choose clothes that are easy to put on.

8. _____ Mark the restroom with a sign as a reminder to use it and where it is.

9. _____ For mealtime, use plain plates with a simple place setting and remove other items from the table.

10. _____ Do not encourage independence as this leads to aggressive behavior.

11. _____ Provide a daily calendar to encourage activities.

12. _____ Monitor weight accurately and frequently.

13. _____ Reward positive behavior with smiles, hugs, warm touches and thank yous.

10. Describe interventions for common difficult behaviors related to Alzheimer's disease

Scenarios.
Read each of the following scenarios involving residents with Alzheimer's disease and answer the questions that follow.

1. Dana is a nursing assistant who has just started working at Parkwood Nursing Home. She is assigned to give Mr. Bruner, a resident with Alzheimer's disease, a bath and a back rub. When Dana meets Mr. Bruner, he gets very upset and yells at Dana to leave him alone. What can Dana do to lessen Mr. Bruner's agitation?

_____

_____

_____

_____

_____

_____

_____

2. Mr. Aaronson, another resident at Parkwood, is upset because he has just found out that his daughter is moving out of the state and will not be able to visit him as often. While watching television in the common area with other residents, he gets angry at Mrs. Robinson for changing the channel. He starts shouting at her and threatens to hit her if she doesn't stop irritating him. How should Dana respond to this behavior?

_____

_____

_____

_____

_____

_____

_____

3. Dana notices that one of her residents, Mr. Boyd, has seemed withdrawn lately and has not been eating as much as usual. He has

lost interest in his treasured book collection and has not wanted to spend any time with his friends or family when they visit. What can Dana do?

_____

_____

_____

_____

_____

_____

_____

4. When Dana arrives at work one morning, she gets several complaints from her residents that Mr. Bruner has been scratching his groin area in the dining room during breakfast and making the other residents at his table uncomfortable. What are some possible causes for this behavior, and how should Dana react?

_____

_____

_____

_____

_____

_____

5. Ms. Stryker is a cheerful, vivacious resident with Alzheimer's disease. She loves to dress in brightly colored clothes and wear tasteful jewelry. Lately she has begun to pick up other residents' clothing and jewelry from their rooms and putting it into her dresser drawer. Her family is very upset by this behavior. What should Dana tell them and how can she help?

_____

_____

_____

_____

_____

_____

_____

_____

_____

_____

_____

_____

11. Discuss ways to provide activities for residents with Alzheimer's disease

True or False.

1. T F Residents with Alzheimer's disease usually do not usually enjoy participating in activities.

2. T F Information from a resident's family should be used to plan activities for him.

3. T F Meaningful activities for a resident with AD draw on past skills that the resident has used throughout his life.

4. T F "Doing" activities will keep a resident with Alzheimer's focused for several hours at a time.

5. T F If a resident loses interest in an activity, the staff should push her to continue until she is finished.

6. T F Residents' families should be encouraged to participate in activities.

7. T F Residents with AD should be discouraged from exercising.

8. T F Each resident should be encouraged to use his or her special skills.

9. T F Reading and playing music are good ways to provide activity for bed-bound residents.

Name: _____

12. Describe therapies for residents with Alzheimer's disease

Matching.

a. Reminiscence therapy

b. Validation therapy

c. Remotivation therapy

d. Reality orientation

1. _____ Type of therapy that promotes self-esteem, self-awareness, and socialization in groups

2. _____ Type of therapy that lets people with Alzheimer's disease believe they live in the past or in imaginary circumstances

3. _____ Type of therapy that encourages people with Alzheimer's disease to remember and talk about the past

4. _____ Type of therapy that uses calendars, clocks, signs, and lists to help people with Alzheimer's disease remember who and where they are

13. Discuss mental health, mental illness, and related disorders

Word Search.
Write the correct word in each blank and find your answers in the word search.

1. _____ _____ is a person's ability to use cognition and emotion appropriately.

2. Mental illness is a _____ that affects a person's ability to function in family, home, work or community settings.

3. _____ is uneasiness or fear about a situation or condition.

4. _____ _____ _____ is characterized by chronic anxiety, excessive worrying, and tension even when there is no cause for these feelings.

5. A person who has had a traumatic experience such as being a victim of a crime or a severe accident may develop _____ _____ _____.

6. Obsessive-compulsive disorder is characterized by _____ behavior used to cope with anxiety.

7. _____ _____ disorder causes extreme self-consciousness in everyday situations and may cause a person to avoid being around other people.

8. Symptoms of _____ disorder include dizziness, rapid heartbeat, upset stomach and a feeling of doom.

9. _____ _____ is a serious mental illness in which a feeling of overwhelming sadness makes it difficult for a person to function normally.

10. If a resident makes comments or jokes about _____ himself, report it immediately to the nurse.

11. A person with _____ _____ may have mood swings and changes in energy level and ability to function.

12. Symptoms of _____ may include hallucinations, delusions, and disorganized thinking and speech.

13. A person with paranoid schizophrenia may experience delusions of _____.

```
f r b t b c b g a q e w r g
u e x j i l i i b d s n r e
w d d r p i a m j w a e o n
b r t n o n h e f g t o q e
v o u j l i x c u d i k f r
p s p e a c x w i r o o j a
n i n s r a d s p n r l n l
l d a k d l x p q e y o h i
k s d n i d m a k s i g k z
w s d w s e g n i t r u h e
a e t e o p t i u q o h b d
y r s z r r e c g a b o t a
y t k a d e e f u c b d w n
o s x f e s z p d w r m j x
r c h c r s n r c v e l b i
z i g e w i i r m n p u g e
r t p j a o n d t m e f u t
j a k i c n s a b u t n g y
l m v h r y l e u r i v g d
t u l t y h g j w c t q b i
s a i n e r h p o z i h c s
a r s a l u j m i c v c q o
y t l b y v b s a t e e a r
l t t v o p m m i i c h c d
h s r j n m q i t y c u v e
s o c i a l a n x i e t y r
i p k t p g u g j l f f a h
n z z w r l d w i i y i v r
w x a n h a u b f w p v q w
g f v i y h h e u s m j d d
```

14. Discuss substance abuse and list signs of substance abuse to report

Short Answer.

1. Define substance abuse.

_____

_____

_____

_____

_____

2. List three risk factors for substance abuse.

_____

_____

_____

_____

_____

_____

3. Under what circumstances is an elderly person more at risk for substance abuse?

_____

_____

_____

_____

_____

_____

_____

Name: _____

23
The Endocrine System

1. Review the key terms in Learning Objective 1 before completing the workbook exercises

2. Explain the structure and function of the endocrine system

Fill in the Blank.
Write the correct answers in the blanks below.

1. Glands produce and secrete chemicals called _____.

2. Testosterone is produced within the _____.

3. The endocrine system is made up of _____ in different areas of the body.

4. The endocrine system influences growth and _____, regulates levels of _____ in the blood, and regulates the ability to _____.

5. The _____ gland, or master gland, controls hormone production of other glands.

6. During stressful situations, _____ and the less potent noradrenaline increase the efficiency of muscle contractions, increase _ _____ rate and blood pressure, and increase blood _____ levels to provide extra energy.

7. The pancreas produces _____, which regulates the amount of glucose available to the cells for _____ .

3. Discuss changes in the endocrine system due to aging

True or False.
Circle the "T" for true or the "F" for false for each statement below.

1. T F   Menopause is a normal change of aging.

2. T F   As men age, testosterone production stops.

3. T F   Insulin production increases with age.

4. T F   As a person gets older, the body is less able to handle stress.

4. Discuss common disorders of the endocrine system

Matching.
For each of the following descriptions, write the letter of the disorder or treatment referred to.

a. Diabetes mellitus

b. Diabetic peripheral neuropathy

c. Diabetic retinopathy

d. Goiter

e. Hyperthyroidism

f. Hypoglycemia

g. Hypothyroidism

h. Polydipsia

i. Polyphagia

j. Polyuria

k. Pre-diabetes

l. Type 1 diabetes

m. Type 2 diabetes

120

Name: _____

1. ____ Insulin reaction; a complication of diabetes that can be life-threatening

2. ____ Condition in which the thyroid produces too much thyroid hormone, causing body processes to speed up

3. ____ Glucose levels are elevated but not high enough to establish diagnosis of diabetes; may cause damage to organs

4. ____ Excessive hunger; possible signal of diabetes

5. ____ Enlarged thyroid

6. ____ Condition in which the pancreas does not produce insulin or produce enough insulin

7. ____ Causes numbness, pain, or tingling of the legs and/or feet and nerve damage over time

8. ____ Causes damage to blood vessels in the eyes; can cause blindness

9. ____ Most common form of diabetes

10. ____ Condition in which the body lacks thyroid hormone, causing body processes to slow down

11. ____ Excessive urination; possible signal of diabetes

12. ____ Formerly known as juvenile diabetes

13. ____ Excessive thirst; possible signal of diabetes

5. Describe care guidelines for diabetes

True or False.

1. T F If you notice any foot problems, such as a rash or fungus on a diabetic resident's foot, wait a day to report it to see if it gets worse.

2. T F Meals must be served at the same time every day for a resident with diabetes.

3. T F If your resident with diabetes is not following her diet, report it to your supervisor.

4. T F Always check the expiration date of test strips for blood glucose monitoring.

5. T F A small sore on a diabetic resident does not need to be reported.

6. T F Nursing assistants should never cut a diabetic resident's toenails.

7. T F Diabetic residents should be discouraged from exercising.

8. T F Diabetic residents should go barefoot to improve circulation in the feet.

6. Discuss foot care guidelines for diabetes

Word Search.
Fill in the correct words in the blanks below, then find your answers in the word search.

1. Diabetes weakens the _____ system, which reduces resistance to _____.

2. Poor _____ due to narrowing of _____ _____ increases chances of infection.

3. When foot infections are not caught early, _____ of a toe, foot, or leg may be necessary.

4. Foot care should be a part of _____ _____ of residents.

5. Avoid _____ soaps and _____ water.

6. Do not use any _____ to try to remove dirt from a toenail.

7. Use a doctor-recommended _____ or _____ on the feet, but never use _____.

8. Remind resident not to walk around _____.

9. Notify the nurse if resident has excessive _____ of the skin of the feet, _____

nails, or change in color of the skin or nails, especially _____.

```
f q k u k n o y c a u b l m
j b t j p g y x t y l h q k
c i r c u l a t i o n w u t
p y r x w i i j o d h o b i
v f f b j n r d h a r s h x
p u b c h f v b d i o g j x
o g n i n e k c a l b n t x
w m g n s c k u o y n i j n
d e s s o t e t z c d n c k
e v e s c i i l a a l g q k
r l c e e o t m q r a r r l
s k j g n n b a r e f o o t
r b u o m s y e t n c w e s
o k l c e q a r v u x n x y
a u f p n b f c d m p i l g
z g m c x k m u y m f m j m
d b a e c d w p g i s g a n
v k g g x a n i v t h k u n
```

24
The Immune and Lymphatic Systems and Cancer

1. Review the key terms in Learning Objective 1 before completing the workbook exercises

2. Explain the structure and function of the immune and lymphatic systems

Fill in the Blank.
Write the correct answers in the blanks below.

1. The clear yellowish fluid that moves into the lymph system and carries disease-fighting cells, lymphocytes, is called

_____.

2. The lymphatic system is composed of lymph, lymph vessels, lymph _____, the spleen, and the _____ gland.

3. A main function of the spleen is to serve as a storage shed for _____.

4. The immune system protects the body from disease-causing _____, _____, and _____.

5. _____ immunity is present at birth; _____ immunity is acquired by the body.

6. In _____ immunity, the body manufactures antibodies as a response to an antigen; with

_____ immunity, a person is given the antibodies needed to defend against the antigen.

3. Discuss changes in the immune and lymphatic systems due to aging

True or False.
Circle the "T" for true or the "F" for false.

1. T F Infections and illnesses may increase with age.

2. T F Vaccines are just as effective for older people as they are for younger people.

3. T F Antibody response speeds up with age.

4. T F T-cells decrease in number as a person gets older.

4. Describe the most common disorder of the immune system

Short Answer.
Write the correct answer to each question below in the space provided.

1. If you had just met someone and she told you she had AIDS, how would you feel?

_____
_____
_____
_____
_____
_____
_____
_____
_____
_____

2. Resident Jeremy Lewis sees you in the hall. He looks upset. He tells you that he accidentally touched another resident with AIDS. He says that he is very worried that he will now "catch it" himself. How do you respond?

_____

124

Name: _____

_____

_____

_____

_____

_____

_____

3. How does HIV harm the body?

_____

_____

_____

_____

_____

_____

4. List three high-risk behaviors that can spread HIV/AIDS.

_____

_____

_____

_____

_____

_____

5. List four common activities that do not spread HIV.

_____

_____

_____

_____

_____

_____

6. What is an opportunistic infection?

_____

_____

_____

_____

5. Discuss infection control guidelines for a resident with HIV/AIDS

Multiple Choice.
Circle the letter of the correct answer.

1. Infection control guidelines for HIV/AIDS include:
    a. Always follow infection control procedures and Standard Precautions with all residents.
    b. Re-cap sharps after use.
    c. It's all right to share personal items if both residents are already infected.
    d. A nursing assistant's supervisor should never be told if the NA has HIV/AIDS.

2. Confidentiality is especially important to people with HIV/AIDS because:
    a. A person with HIV/AIDS can be fired from their job.
    b. Others may pass judgment on people with this disease.
    c. A person can be forced to be tested for HIV.
    d. A healthcare worker with HIV/AIDS is not at risk of acquiring infections from patients.

6. Discuss care guidelines for a resident with HIV/AIDS

Crossword Puzzle.
Fill in the correct word in each blank below and use your answers to complete the crossword puzzle.

Across.

3. Special _____ may be ordered to assist with maintaining or gaining weight.

7. Some people may avoid a person with AIDS due to _____, or a fear of homosexuality.

8. Protect the resident from people having known _____ diseases.

9. Encourage resident to be as

_____

   as possible.

12. Use special soft _____
    or swabs when cleaning the mouth and per-
    forming oral care.

13. Perform _____ _____

    _____

    exercises as ordered.

14. Allow enough rest and recognize

    _____.

Down.

1. HIV- or AIDS-infected persons may not be
   able to be around _____
   due to the risk of different types of
   infection.

2. Spend _____
   time with residents who have HIV or AIDS.

4. Monitor vital signs often, especially

   _____.

5. Notify the nurse of any

   _____

   that puts the resident or others at risk.

6. Helping residents with HIV or AIDS avoid
   _____ is
   important.

10. Give _____
    support as well as physical care.

11. Observe the skin closely for skin

    _____.

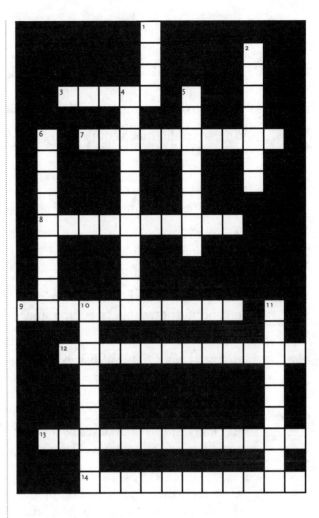

7. Describe cancer

Matching.
*For each description, write in the letter of the correct
term.*

a. Benign

b. Biopsy

c. Cancer

d. Chemotherapy

e. Hormone therapy

f. Immunotherapy

g. Malignant

h. Metastasize

i. Oncology

j. Palliative care

k. Radiotherapy

l. Remission

m. Surgery

n. Tumor

1. ____ Non-cancerous

2. ____ A group of abnormally-growing cells

3. ____ Spread to other areas of the body

4. ____ Cancerous

5. ____ Type of care that works to relieve symptoms and reduce pain and suffering

6. ____ Reduction in or disappearance of signs and symptoms of cancer

7. ____ Can be effective when tumors rely on specific hormones to survive and grow

8. ____ Removal of a sample of tissue for examination and diagnosis

9. ____ One form is a cancer vaccine

10. ____ General term used to describe a disease in which abnormal cells grow in an uncontrolled way

11. ____ Uses high-energy rays to attempt to destroy cancer cells in a specific area

12. ____ Branch of medicine that deals with study and treatment of cancer

13. ____ Goal is to remove as much of the cancer as possible

14. ____ Chemical agents or medications are administered to kill malignant cells and tissues

8. Discuss care guidelines for a resident with cancer

Short Answer.
For each of the following concerns for a resident with cancer, write one reason why it is important.

1. Skin care

_____

_____

_____

_____

2. Self-image

_____

_____

_____

_____

3. Oral care

_____

_____

_____

_____

4. Pain management

_____

_____

_____

_____

5. Vital signs

_____

_____

_____

_____

6. Mobility

_____

_____

_____

_____

7. Nutrition

_____

_____

_____

_____

8. Bladder and bowel changes

_____

_____

Name: _____

_____

_____

9. Mental status and emotional needs

_____

_____

_____

_____

Name: _____

25
Rehabilitation and Restorative Care

1. Review the key terms in Learning Objective 1 before completing the workbook exercises

2. Discuss rehabilitation and restorative care

Short Answer.
Write the correct answer to each question below in the space provided.

1. Define rehabilitation.

   _____

   _____

   _____

   _____

2. List three goals of rehabilitative care.

   _____

   _____

   _____

   _____

   _____

   _____

3. In what ways are nursing assistants vital to the rehabilitation team?

   _____

   _____

   _____

   _____

3. Describe the importance of promoting independence

True or False.
Circle the "T" for true or the "F" for false.

1. T F Being able to perform activities of daily living is not very important.

2. T F Dressing is an example of an ADL.

3. T F Being required to accept help with ADLs can cause a decrease in the resident's abilities.

4. T F If a resident is doing a task too slowly, a nursing assistant should offer to do it for her.

5. T F Independence helps with self-esteem and can help speed recovery.

6. T F Verbal and physical cues are not usually helpful during rehabilitative care.

7. T F Residents have a legal right to make choices about food, doctors, and how to spend their time.

4. Explain the complications of immobility and describe how exercise helps maintains health

Short Answer.
For each of these body systems, write one benefit of regular activity: integumentary system, musculoskeletal system, circulatory system, respiratory system, gastrointestinal system, urinary system, and nervous system.

   _____

   _____

   _____

   _____

   _____

   _____

Name: _____

_____
_____
_____
_____
_____
_____
_____

5. Describe canes, walkers and crutches

Multiple Choice.
Circle the letter of the correct answer.

1. When using a cane, how should a resident move?
    a. Cane first, strong leg, then weak leg
    b. Weak leg, strong leg, then cane
    c. Strong leg, cane, then weak leg
    d. Cane, weak leg, then strong leg

2. Walking aids include all of the following EXCEPT:
    a. Wheelchair
    b. Cane
    c. Walker
    d. Crutches

3. Which of the following walking aids are used when a resident can only bear limited weight or cannot bear any weight at all on one leg?
    a. C-cane
    b. Quad cane
    c. Walker
    d. Crutches

4. All of the following are guidelines for use of canes, walkers and crutches EXCEPT:
    a. Check device for any damage before using.
    b. Watch for and avoid unsafe environmental situations.
    c. When resident is ambulating, stay near the resident's stronger side.
    d. Do not rush the resident.

6. Discuss other assistive devices or orthotics

Fill in the Blank.
Fill in the correct word in each blank below.

1. Assistive or _____ devices can help people who are recovering from illness or adapting to a disability.

2. _____ _____ is a weakness of muscles in the feet and ankles that interferes with the ability to walk normally.

3. _____ or hip wedges keep hips in proper position after hip surgery.

4. Trochanter rolls prevent the hip and leg from turning _____.

5. Handrolls help prevent finger, hand, or wrist _____.

7. Discuss range of motion exercises

Matching.
For each description, write the letter of the correct term in the blank.

a. Abduction

b. Active assisted range of motion (AAROM)

c. Active range of motion (AROM)

d. Adduction

e. Dorsiflexion

f. Extension

g. Flexion

h. Passive range of motion (PROM)

i. Pronation

j. Range of motion exercises

k. Rotation

l. Supination

1. ____ Done by resident with some help from a staff member

2. ____ Straightening a body part

3. ____ Exercises that put a joint through its full arc of motion

4. ____ Turning downward

5. ____ Moving a body part away from the midline of the body

6. ____ Done by staff without resident's help

7. ____ Turning upward

8. ____ Done by a resident alone, without help

9. ____ Moving a body part toward the midline of the body

10. ____ Bending backward

11. ____ Bending a body part

12. ____ Turning the joint

Name: _____

26
Subacute Care

1. Review the key terms in Learning Objective 1 before completing the workbook exercises

2. Discuss the types of residents who are in a subacute setting

Short Answer.
Answer each question below in the space provided.

1. What is subacute care, and where is it usually provided?

_____

_____

_____

_____

_____

_____

_____

_____

_____

2. List five conditions that might call for subacute care.

_____

_____

_____

_____

_____

_____

_____

_____

_____

_____

3. List care guidelines for pulse oximetry

True or False.
Circle the "T" for true or the "F" for false.

1. T F A pulse oximeter measures a person's blood oxygen level and pulse rate.

2. T F Generally, a normal blood oxygen level is less than 90%.

3. T F Diseases such as COPD can lower a person's blood oxygen level.

4. T F If the alarm on the pulse oximeter sounds, the nursing assistant should turn it off.

4. Describe telemetry and list care guidelines

Fill in the Blank.
Fill in the correct work in each blank below.

1. Telemetry is the application of a

_____

monitoring device.

2. The telemetry unit transmits information about the heart's _____ and _____ to a central monitoring station.

3. A portable telemetry unit attaches to a resident's _____.

4. Monitor _____ _____ carefully as ordered.

5. Report if pads become _____.

6. Report to the nurse if patient has chest pain or _____, rapid _____, or shortness of _____.

Name: _____

5. Explain artificial airways and list care guidelines

Multiple Choice.
Circle the letter of the correct answer.

1. An artificial airway may be needed due to blockage caused by all of the following EXCEPT:
   a. Illness
   b. Secretions
   c. Tachycardia
   d. Aspiration

2. A surgically created opening in the neck into the trachea is called a(n):
   a. Intubation
   b. Stoma
   c. Trach tube
   d. Tracheostomy

3. All of the following are guidelines for artificial airways EXCEPT:
   a. Oral care should not be performed on residents with artificial airways.
   b. Use other methods of communication, such as writing notes or communication boards, if resident cannot speak.
   c. Be supportive and encouraging.
   d. Notify the nurse of wheezing or other unusual breathing sounds, secretions in tubing, or cyanosis.

6. Discuss care for a resident with a tracheostomy

Crossword Puzzle.
Fill in the correct answers in the blanks below, then use your answers to complete the crossword puzzle.

Across.

3. General tracheostomy care includes keeping the skin around the opening, or

   _____, clean.

5. A tracheostomy may be necessary due to serious _____ reactions.

7. A _____
   is a common type of artificial airway seen in long-term care.

11. Do not _____
   tracheostomy opening.

12. Be careful to prevent

   _____

   when cleaning the mouth.

13. _____
   may be needed frequently with this type of resident.

Down.

1. Report change in vital signs, especially

   _____ _____.

2. Answer _____ _____ promptly.

4. Careful _____ and
   reporting by nursing assistants is vital.

6. _____ boards
   can be used if the resident cannot speak.

8. Do not move or remove spare tracheostomy tubes or spare bag _____

   _____.

9. While the tracheostomy is in place, the resident may not be able to

   _____.

10. Assist resident to get into the ordered

   _____.

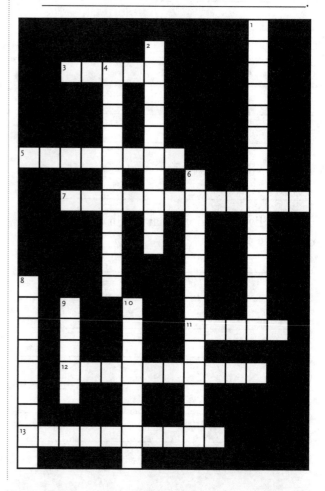

7. Describe mechanical ventilation and explain care guidelines

True or False.

1. T F A ventilator performs the process of breathing for a person who cannot breathe on his own.

2. T F Residents on a ventilator are usually able to speak clearly.

3. T F Residents on a ventilator will usually prefer to be left alone as much as possible.

4. T F Residents on a ventilator are often heavily sedated.

5. T F A resident on a ventilator needs to be positioned flat on his back at all times.

6. T F Reposition the resident at least every two hours.

7. T F Residents on ventilators will require one-on-one care during a power failure.

8. T F Most residents on ventilators will show nervousness or anxiety, so it is not necessary to notify the nurse if this occurs.

9. T F Symptoms of severe sepsis include chills, weakness, headache, and confusion.

8. Describe suctioning and list signs of respiratory distress

Short Answer.

1. When is suctioning needed?

_____

_____

_____

_____

2. List four signs of respiratory distress.

_____

_____

_____

3. List six guidelines for suctioning.

_____

_____

_____

_____

_____

_____

_____

_____

_____

_____

9. Describe chest tubes and explain related care

Word Search.
Fill in the correct word in each blank below, then find your answers in the word search.

1. Chest tubes are _____ drainage tubes that are inserted into the chest during a sterile procedure.

2. Chest tubes are used to drain air, pus, blood, or _____ that has collected in the _____ cavity or to allow a full expansion of the _____.

3. Some conditions that require chest tube insertion include _____, or air or gas in the pleural cavity, _____, or blood in the pleural cavity, or chest _____ or injuries.

4. Drainage systems include those using _____ drainage and _____.

Name: _____

5. Always keep the drainage system

_____

the level of the resident's chest.

6. Report signs of respiratory

_____ immediately.

7. Equipment that is kept nearby in case the tube is pulled out includes special _____, clamp, and bottles of _____ fluid.

8. If asked to assist with _____ and _____ _____ exercises, be encouraging and patient.

9. Report any increase or decrease in

_____ in

the drainage system.

```
b f r s q o p d w e w h v h
p v l h y d r e p g o b o r
m w v u t c u o j f q r e n
w v j f i d c k m h a r v b
n d x w v d i k j a n a c d
j e z u a g a s t l o g c v
a z n x r p l u n g s i x n
x h j c g n i l b b u b s w
s h o t o e o m e u c x s h
f h p l e u r a l g t i e b
y f z n l m g g o e i m r h
d c x x i o k h w g o v t d
a m u a r t w y i t n b s c
k d y o e h z t h n o g i c
d d p d t o f o u i g y d r
i m n b s r r x p b p p a i
g n i h t a e r b p e e d r
a i b s x x f u n a n s k i
```

10. Describe alternative feeding methods and related care

Matching.

a. Central venous line

b. Feeding pump

c. Gastric suctioning

d. Gastrostomy

e. Nasogastric tube

f. Percutaneous Endoscopic Gastrostomy (PEG) Tube

g. Orogastric tube

h. Total parenteral nutrition (TPN)

i. Tube feedings

1. ____ Tube placed through the skin directly into the abdomen

2. ____ Help to regulate the amount of fluid given during tube feeding

3. ____ Tube inserted into the nose for feeding

4. ____ Resident receives nutrients intravenously, bypassing the digestive tract

5. ____ Opening in the stomach and abdomen through which PEG tube is placed

6. ____ Placed in one of the larger veins in the body when TPN is expected to be needed for a while

7. ____ Tube inserted into the mouth for feeding

8. ____ Used for removal by suctioning of materials inside the body

9. ____ Used when residents have swallowing difficulties but can digest food

11. Discuss care guidelines for dialysis

Short Answer.

1. What is kidney dialysis and why is it used?

_____

_____

_____

_____

_____

_____

_____

_____

_____

Name: _____

2. List five things to report to the nurse about dialysis.

_____

_____

_____

_____

_____

_____

_____

27
End-of-Life Care

1. Review the key terms in Learning Objective 1 before completing the workbook exercises

2. Describe palliative care

Short Answer.
Answer the following questions in the space provided.

1. When is palliative care given?

_____
_____
_____
_____
_____

2. List four goals of palliative care.

_____
_____
_____
_____
_____
_____

3. Discuss hospice care

True or False.
Circle the "T" for true or the "F" for false.

1. T F   Hospice care is ordered by a doctor when a person has six months or less to live.

2. T F   Hospice care is not offered on Sundays.

3. T F   Hospice care focuses on curing the resident.

4. T F   In hospice care, it is important to make residents comfortable and manage their pain rather than trying to help them recover.

5. T F   Hospice care uses a holistic approach.

4. Discuss the grief process and related terms

Multiple Choice.
Circle the letter of the correct answer.

1. Mr. Anderson, a resident, talks to God about his terminal cancer. He promises to make peace with his estranged son if he is allowed to live. Which stage of dying is Mr. Anderson going through?
    a. Denial
    b. Anger
    c. Bargaining
    d. Depression
    e. Acceptance

2. Luke, a nursing assistant, knows that his resident, Ms. Wilson, is dying. One day Ms. Wilson begins to yell at Luke, blaming him for a lack of proper care, saying, "If you had been a better caregiver, I would never have gotten sick." Luke tries to comfort her, not taking it personally because he realizes that this is the _____ stage of dying.
    a. Denial
    b. Anger
    c. Bargaining
    d. Depression
    e. Acceptance

3. Mrs. Morris is a resident who is dying. She has an appointment with her attorney. When he visits her in her room, he says, "I just want to make sure everything is in order with your will." She thanks him nicely but tells him she has no idea why he would want to talk about that subject. Instead she wants

to talk about her son. Which stage of dying is Mrs. Morris in?

a. Denial
b. Anger
c. Bargaining
d. Depression
e. Acceptance

4. Gwen, a nursing assistant, notices that her resident, Wes, seems a little distant. When he talks to her, he only wants to discuss the specifics of his funeral arrangements. He is very concerned about making sure his family is taken care of after he is gone. Gwen takes notes on everything he says. In which stage of dying is Wes?

a. Denial
b. Anger
c. Bargaining
d. Depression
e. Acceptance

5. Angelica, a nursing assistant, is worried about one of her terminally ill residents. He alternates between crying and not talking. This resident is experiencing _____.

a. Denial
b. Anger
c. Bargaining
d. Depression
e. Acceptance

5. Explain the dying person's rights

Short Answer.
For each of the rights of a dying person listed below, write one way that a nursing assistant can honor that right.

1. The right to have visitors

_____

_____

_____

_____

2. The right to privacy

_____

_____

3. The right to be free from pain

_____

_____

_____

_____

4. The right to honest and accurate information

_____

_____

_____

_____

5. The right to refuse treatment

_____

_____

_____

_____

_____

6. Explain how to care for a dying resident

Fill in the Blank.
Mark an "X" by each suggestion below that is a good idea for caring for a dying resident.

1. _____ Use alternative methods of communication if speech fails

2. _____ Stop talking to resident as he is probably unaware of his surroundings

3. _____ Keep room softly lit

4. _____ Turn and position resident frequently

5. _____ Change gowns and sheets often

6. _____ Feed resident quickly

Name: _____

7. _____ Observe resident for signs of pain

8. _____ Force resident to eat and drink

9. _____ Clean up for incontinent resident promptly

7. Discuss factors that influence feelings about death and list ways to meet residents' individual needs

Short Answer.

1. Briefly describe how your culture or another culture that you are familiar with responds to death.

_____

_____

_____

_____

_____

_____

_____

_____

_____

_____

2. Have you ever experienced the death of a loved one? If so, how did you grieve?

_____

_____

_____

_____

_____

_____

_____

_____

_____

_____

3. List seven guidelines for meeting the psychosocial and spiritual needs of a dying resident.

_____

_____

_____

_____

_____

_____

_____

_____

_____

_____

_____

_____

_____

_____

_____

_____

8. Identify common signs of approaching death

Fill in the Blank.
Mark an "X" beside the signs of approaching death.

1. _____ high blood pressure

2. _____ fever

3. _____ cold, pale skin

4. _____ confusion

5. _____ healthy skin tone

6. _____ heightened sense of touch

7. _____ inability to speak

8. _____ incontinence

9. _____ perspiration

10. _____ quick, regular breaths

Name: _____

9. List changes that may occur in the human body after death

Fill in the Blank.
Write the correct word in each blank.

1. When death occurs, the body will not have a
   _____, pulse,
   respiration, or _____ _____.

2. The _____ drops, caus-
   ing the mouth to stay _____.

3. _____ may be partially open
   with eyes in a _____ _____.

4. Resident may be incontinent of both
   _____ and
   _____.

5. The pupils will be _____
   and _____.

6. If you see any of these signs, tell the nurse
   so that She will _____
   _ the death.

10. Describe ways to help family and friends deal with a resident's death

True or False.

1. T F If a family member becomes very
   angry with you after a loved one's
   death, it is a good idea to try to calm
   her down.

2. T F Family and friends may feel guilt
   after a loved one's death, especially if
   there were unresolved issues in the
   relationship.

3. T F It is not normal for family and
   friends to have a feeling of relief after
   a loved one has died.

4. T F Let family members and friends talk
   about their feelings.

5. T F Do not allow residents' family and
   friends to know that you are upset
   about the death of a resident.

6. T F Reassuring family and friends that
   they will get over the death of their
   loved one is helpful.

11. Describe ways to help staff members cope with a resident's death

Word Search.
Fill in the correct word in each blank below and find your answers in the word search.

1. Being able to _____ is important.

2. Some facilities offer
   _____ _____
   to help staff with grieving.

3. Many facilities allow caregivers and residents to participate in _____
   or _____ services following
   a death.

4. Do not be _____ because
   you feel grief about the death of a resident.

5. _____ and _____
   are normal responses to grieving.

6. Do things that make you _____
   and spend _____ time with
   people you love.

7. Join a special _____
   _____ for grieving.

b	c	r	y	i	n	g	v	h	v	z	t	v	v
s	u	p	p	o	r	t	g	r	o	u	p	s	b
a	s	h	a	m	e	d	t	m	n	k	r	e	h
d	s	b	r	n	l	a	y	s	l	y	m	k	s
n	t	x	e	b	i	m	t	a	m	s	r	m	c
e	p	h	h	f	g	r	i	e	v	e	o	n	i
s	v	v	t	p	i	r	l	t	r	y	p	w	k
s	x	m	t	g	o	l	a	q	e	s	q	m	o
d	q	p	n	m	u	u	u	e	b	r	o	p
q	q	y	e	z	s	h	q	o	t	c	s	e	k
w	f	m	m	l	n	a	r	n	i	y	z	m	x
x	o	z	e	e	f	f	i	n	g	e	o	k	y
n	m	f	v	h	f	q	p	t	f	c	z	k	a
u	x	y	a	n	d	w	p	m	t	s	b	b	m
b	k	p	e	j	w	b	n	f	h	d	i	w	i
h	p	g	r	f	c	u	s	c	y	z	a	n	r
y	e	r	e	h	p	v	m	v	g	b	k	j	a
i	l	z	b	c	j	r	n	z	k	s	f	u	q

12. Describe postmortem care

Short Answer.

1. Define "postmortem care."

    _____
    _____
    _____
    _____
    _____
    _____
    _____

2. What is the purpose of an autopsy?

    _____
    _____
    _____
    _____
    _____
    _____
    _____

3. What should a nursing assistant do after the body has been transported?

    _____
    _____
    _____
    _____

28
Your New Position

1. Review the key terms in Learning Objective 1 before completing the workbook exercises

2. Describe how to write a résumé and cover letter

True or False.
Circle "T" for true or "F" for false for each statement below.

1. T F   You should explain your entire work history in your cover letter.

2. T F   You should not list your education on your résumé.

3. T F   The first step in any job search is to prepare a résumé.

4. T F   A résumé should be at least three pages long.

5. T F   A cover letter should include information on why you are seeking the job and why you are qualified for the position.

3. Identify information that may be required for filling out a job application

Short Answer.
Answer the following questions in the space provided.

1. List six examples of information you might need when filling out a job application.

_____

_____

_____

_____

_____

_____

_____

2. List three guidelines for filling out a job application.

_____

_____

_____

_____

_____

_____

_____

_____

4. Discuss proper grooming guidelines for a job interview

Fill in the Blank.
Write "Yes" or "No" next to the description below to indicate whether it is appropriate preparation for a job interview.

1. _____   Wear rings on every finger.

2. _____   Brush your teeth beforehand.

3. _____   Smoke a cigarette right before the interview to calm down.

4. _____   Do not wear perfume or cologne.

5. _____   Wear jeans.

6. _____   Wear high-heeled black sandals.

5. List techniques for interviewing successfully

Fill in the Blank.
Write "Yes" or "No" next to each behavior below to indicate whether or not it is appropriate for a job interview.

1. _____ Look around the room while you're being interviewed.

2. _____ Shake hands firmly with the interviewer.

3. _____ Practice for the interview.

4. _____ Do not smile.

5. _____ Arrive ten to fifteen minutes early for the interview.

6. _____ Exaggerate your accomplishments.

7. _____ Write a follow-up thank-you letter.

6. Describe a standard job description and list steps for following the scope of practice

Crossword Puzzle.
Fill in the correct words in the blanks below and use your answers to complete the crossword puzzle.

Across.

5. You should _____ the job description before you sign it.

6. A _____ _____ is an outline of what will be expected of you in your job.

8. Do not perform a procedure if you have not been _____ to do it.

9. Do not perform a(n) _____ if it is not listed in your job description.

Down.

1. Doing things beyond your scope of practice could _____ a resident, you, or another staff member.

2. If you do not understand anything on the job description, you should _____ _____.

3. Nursing assistants must follow their _____ _____ _____.

4. Purchasing an inexpensive _____ _____ can help you organize your workdays.

5. If you believe a procedure may not be appropriate for a certain _____, ask the nurse before performing it.

7. Do not perform a procedure if you have _____ how to do it.

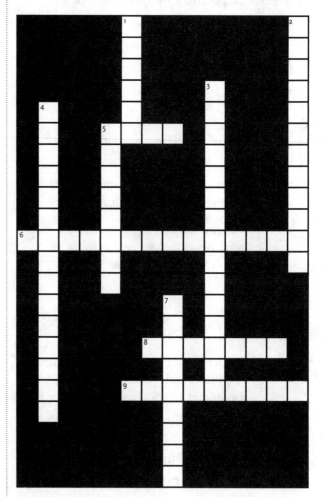

7. Identify guidelines for maintaining certification and explain the state's registry

Multiple Choice.

1. What is the minimum number of hours of training a nursing assistant must complete before being employed, according to OBRA?
   a. 50
   b. 70
   c. 75
   d. 100

2. Within how many months of training must a nursing assistant usually take the state test?
   a. 6 months
   b. 1 year
   c. 18 months
   d. 24 months

3. In most states, a nursing assistant has ____ chance(s) to pass the state test.
   a. One
   b. Two
   c. Three
   d. Four

4. Information kept in the state registry for nursing assistants includes all of the following EXCEPT:
   a. Information about investigations and hearings regarding abuse, neglect, or theft
   b. The nursing assistant's medical records
   c. Expiration dates of nursing assistants' certificates
   d. The nursing assistant's home address, date of birth and social security number

8. Describe continuing education for nursing assistants

True or False.

1. T F OBRA requires that nursing assistants must have 12 hours of continuing education each year in order to keep certification current.

2. T F The continuing education requirement for all states is the same as OBRA's.

3. T F Subjects covered in continuing education include Residents' Rights, infection control, and confidentiality.

4. T F Employers are required to provide free hepatitis B vaccines for all employees, as well as a tuberculosis test once per year.

9. Describe employee evaluations and discuss criticism

Fill in the Blank.

1. An annual _____, sometimes called a performance _____ or review, is used to evaluate the performance of each employee.

2. Employees may be evaluated on overall _____, _____ resolution, and _____ effort.

3. _____ criticism is the process of giving opinions about the work of others, which includes helpful suggestions for change.

4. _____ criticism is angry and negative.

5. When receiving constructive criticism, be _____ to suggestions that will help you _____ and be more _____ in your work.

6. If you are not sure how to avoid a _____ you have made, ask for suggestions.

7. Performance reviews are frequently the basis for _____ _____.

8. A satisfactory review can increase your chances of _____ within the facility.

10. Discuss conflict resolution

Short Answer.

1. What is conflict resolution?

_____

_____

_____

_____

_____

2. What should a nursing assistant always do when changing jobs?

_____

_____

_____

_____

_____

_____

_____

11. Define "stress" and explain ways to manage stress

Matching.
Match each term or list below to the appropriate description.

a. Abdominal breathing

b. Burnout

c. Increasing exercise, developing new hobbies, setting realistic goals

d. Residents and residents' families

e. Smoking, increasing caffeine in diet, taking illegal drugs

f. Stress

g. Stressor

h. Supervisor, doctor, friends and family, spiritual leader

1. ____ An internal or external factor or stimulus that causes stress

2. ____ Mental or physical exhaustion due to a prolonged period of stress and frustration

3. ____ Unhealthy responses to stress

4. ____ A relaxation technique for managing stress

5. ____ Appropriate people to turn to for help with stress

6. ____ Healthy ways to manage stress

7. ____ Inappropriate people to talk to about stress

8. ____ A mentally or emotionally disruptive or upsetting condition that occurs due to changes in the environment

12. Describe how to be a valued member of the healthcare community

Short Answer.

1. Think of two people to thank for helping you to complete your nursing assistant training course.

_____

_____

_____

_____

_____

2. Think of one thing you are going to do to reward yourself for meeting this goal.

_____

_____

_____

_____

_____

3. Think of one thing you will do to keep learning as you move forward in your new profession.

_____

_____

_____

_____

_____

Procedure Checklists

Washing hands

		yes	no
1.	Identifies self by name. Identifies resident. Greets resident by name.		
2.	Turns on water at sink.		
3.	Angles arms downward, with fingertips pointing down and hands lower than elbows. Wets hands and wrists thoroughly.		
4.	Applies skin cleanser or soap to hands.		
5.	Lathers all surfaces of hands, wrists, and fingers, using friction for at least 20 seconds.		
6.	Cleans nails by rubbing fingertips in palm of other hand.		
7.	Rinses all surfaces of wrists, hands, and fingers, keeping hands lower than elbows and fingertips down.		
8.	Uses clean, dry paper towel to dry all surfaces of hands, wrists, and fingers.		
9.	Uses clean, dry paper towel or knee to turn off faucet without contaminating hands.		
10.	Disposes of used paper towels in wastebasket immediately after shutting off faucet.		

_____   _____
Date Reviewed   Instructor Signature

_____   _____
Date Performed   Instructor Signature

Putting on gloves

		yes	no
1.	Washes hands.		
2.	If right-handed, slides one glove onto left hand (reverses if left-handed).		
3.	Using gloved hand, slides other hand into second glove.		
4.	Interlaces fingers to smooth out folds and create a comfortable fit.		
5.	Checks for tears, holes, cracks, or discolored spots in gloves. Replaces gloves if needed.		
6.	Adjusts gloves until they are pulled up over wrist and fit correctly. If wearing gown, pulls cuff of gloves over sleeves of gown.		

_____   _____
Date Reviewed   Instructor Signature

_____   _____
Date Performed   Instructor Signature

Taking off gloves

		yes	no
1.	Touches only outside of one glove. Pulls first glove off by pulling down from cuff toward fingers. Glove comes off turned inside-out.		
2.	With fingertips of gloved hand, holds glove just removed.		
3.	With ungloved hand, reaches two fingers inside remaining glove without touching outside of glove.		

4.	Pulls down, turning glove inside-out and over first glove.		
5.	Drops both gloves into proper container.		
6.	Washes hands.		

_____   _____
Date Reviewed   Instructor Signature

_____   _____
Date Performed   Instructor Signature

Putting on a gown

		yes	no
1.	Washes hands.		
2.	Removes watch and places it on clean paper towel. If wearing long sleeves, pushes or rolls them up.		
3.	Holds gown out front to open it without shaking. Slips arms into sleeves and pulls gown on.		
4.	Securely fastens at neck and waist. Ties neck ties into a bow or seals tapes closed.		
5.	Reaches back and pulls gown until it completely covers clothing. Ties back ties.		

_____   _____
Date Reviewed   Instructor Signature

_____   _____
Date Performed   Instructor Signature

Putting on a mask and goggles

		yes	no
1.	Washes hands.		
2.	Picks up mask by top strings or elastic strap. Does not touch mask where it touches face.		
3.	Adjusts mask over nose and mouth. Ties top strings, then bottom strings. Does not wear mask hanging from bottom strings.		

4.	Pinches metal strip at top of mask tightly around nose and fits mask snugly around face and below chin.		
5.	Puts on goggles and positions them over eyes. Secures them to head using headband or ear-pieces.		
6.	Puts on gloves after putting on mask and goggles.		

_____   _____
Date Reviewed   Instructor Signature

_____   _____
Date Performed   Instructor Signature

Applying and removing the full set of PPE

		yes	no
Applying:			
1.	Washes hands.		
2.	Puts on gown.		
3.	Applies mask or respirator.		
4.	Applies goggles or face shield.		
5.	Applies gloves last.		
Removing:			
1.	Removes gloves first and discards in proper container.		
2.	Washes hands.		
3.	Removes face shield or goggles if used.		
4.	Removes gown and discards in proper container.		
5.	Removes mask or respirator and discards in proper container.		
6.	Washes hands.		

_____   _____
Date Reviewed   Instructor Signature

_____   _____
Date Performed   Instructor Signature

Applying a physical tie restraint safely

		yes	no
1.	Identifies self by name. Identifies resident and greets resident by name.		
2.	Washes hands.		
3.	Explains procedure to resident. Speaks clearly, slowly, and directly. Maintains face-to-face contact whenever possible. Encourages resident to assist if possible.		
4.	Provides for resident's privacy with a curtain, screen, or door.		
5.	Applies restraint carefully, following manufacturer's directions and facility policy, making sure they are not too tight. CHEST or BELT-STYLE RESTRAINTS: Makes sure not to catch breasts or skin in restraints. VEST: Places criss-cross in vest restraint on front of body. MITT: Places a rolled-up washcloth or commercial hand roll in mitt restraint. WRIST/ANKLE: Makes sure restraint will not slide off wrist or ankle.		
6.	Uses slip knot to tie restraint. Makes sure it is not too tight. If restraint is used on a resident who is in bed, ties it to movable part of bed frame.		
7.	Makes resident comfortable.		
8.	Leaves call light within resident's reach.		
9.	Washes hands.		
10.	Is courteous and respectful at all times.		
11.	Reports any changes to nurse and documents procedure using facility guidelines.		

_____   _____
Date Reviewed   Instructor Signature

_____   _____
Date Performed   Instructor Signature

Abdominal thrusts for the conscious person

		yes	no
1.	Stands behind person, bringing arms under resident's arms. Wraps arms around person's waist.		
2.	Makes a fist with one hand and places flat, thumb side of fist against person's abdomen, above navel but below breastbone.		
3.	Grasps fist with other hand and pulls both hands toward self and up, quickly and forcefully.		
4.	Repeats until object is pushed out or person loses consciousness.		

_____   _____
Date Reviewed   Instructor Signature

_____   _____
Date Performed   Instructor Signature

Shock

		yes	no
1.	Notifies nurse immediately.		
2.	Controls bleeding.		
3.	Has person lie down on back unless there is bleeding from mouth or vomiting.		
4.	Checks pulse and respirations if possible. Begins CPR if breathing or pulse is absent.		
5.	Keeps person as calm and comfortable as possible. Loosens clothing or ties around neck and any belts or waist strings.		

6.	Maintains normal body temperature.		
7.	Elevates feet unless person has a head, neck or abdominal injury, breathing difficulties, or a fractured bone or back.		
8.	Does not give person anything to eat or drink.		

_____   _____
Date Reviewed   Instructor Signature

_____   _____
Date Performed   Instructor Signature

Bleeding

		yes	no
1.	Notifies nurse immediately.		
2.	Puts on gloves.		
3.	Holds thick sterile pad, clean pad or clean cloth against wound.		
4.	Presses down hard directly on bleeding wound until help arrives. Does not decrease pressure. Puts additional pads over first pad if blood seeps through; does not remove first pad.		
5.	If able, raises wound above level of heart.		
6.	When bleeding is under control, secures dressing. Checks person for symptoms of shock. Stays with person until help arrives.		
7.	Removes gloves and washes hands thoroughly.		

_____   _____
Date Reviewed   Instructor Signature

_____   _____
Date Performed   Instructor Signature

Burns

		yes	no
For a minor burn:			
1.	Notifies nurse immediately.		

2.	Uses cool, clean water (not ice) to decrease skin temperature and prevent further injury.		
3.	Dampens a clean cloth and places it over burn.		
4.	Covers area with dry, sterile gauze.		
For more serious burns:			
1.	Removes person from source of burn.		
2.	Notifies nurse immediately.		
3.	Checks for breathing, pulse, and severe bleeding.		
4.	Removes as much clothing around burned area as possible. Does not try to pull away clothing that sticks to burn. Covers burn with thick, dry, sterile gauze or a clean cloth.		
5.	Asks person to lie down. Elevates affected part if this does not cause greater pain.		
6.	If burn covers a larger area, wraps person or limb in a dry, clean sheet.		
7.	Waits for emergency medical help.		

_____   _____
Date Reviewed   Instructor Signature

_____   _____
Date Performed   Instructor Signature

Fainting

		yes	no
1.	Notifies or has someone notify nurse immediately.		
2.	Has person lie down or sit down before fainting occurs.		
3.	If person is in sitting position, has her bend forward and place her head between her knees. If person is lying flat on her back, elevates legs.		
4.	Loosens any tight clothing.		

5.	Has person stay in position for at least five minutes after symptoms disappear.		
6.	Helps person get up slowly and continues to observe for symptoms of fainting. Assists her to sit down if needed. Stays with her until she feels better.		

Date Reviewed   Instructor Signature

Date Performed   Instructor Signature

Poisoning

		yes	no
1.	Notifies nurse immediately.		
2.	Puts on gloves. Looks for a container to determine what resident has taken or eaten. With gloves on, opens mouth and looks inside to check mouth for chemical burns. Does not place fingers inside mouth. Notes breath odor.		
3.	Calls Poison Control Center if directed by nurse. Follows their instructions.		

Date Reviewed   Instructor Signature

Date Performed   Instructor Signature

Nosebleed

		yes	no
1.	Notifies nurse immediately.		
2.	Elevates head of bed. Tells resident to remain in sitting position. Offers tissues or clean cloth.		
3.	Puts on gloves. Applies firm pressure over bridge of nose. Squeezes bridge of nose with thumb and forefinger.		
4.	Applies pressure until bleeding stops.		

5.	Uses a cool cloth or ice wrapped in a cloth on back of neck, forehead, or upper lip to slow blood flow.		
6.	Keeps person still and calm until help arrives.		

Date Reviewed   Instructor Signature

Date Performed   Instructor Signature

Vomiting

		yes	no
1.	Notifies nurse immediately.		
2.	Puts on gloves.		
3.	Places an emesis basin under chin. Removes it when vomiting has stopped.		
4.	Provides comfort to resident. Wipes his face and mouth. Provides oral care.		
5.	Removes soiled linens or clothes and replaces with fresh ones.		
6.	If resident's intake and output (I&O) is being monitored, measures and notes amount of vomitus.		
7.	Flushes vomit down toilet and washes and stores basin. Puts soiled linen in proper containers.		
8.	Removes gloves.		
9.	Washes hands again.		
10.	Documents time, amount, color, odor and consistency of vomitus. Observes for blood and reports changes to nurse.		

Date Reviewed   Instructor Signature

Date Performed   Instructor Signature

Myocardial infarction

		yes	no
1.	Calls or has someone call nurse.		
2.	Places resident in a comfortable position and encourages him to rest. Reassures him that he will not be left alone.		
3.	Loosens clothing around neck.		
4.	Does not give resident liquids or food.		
5.	Monitors resident's breathing and pulse. If resident stops breathing or has no pulse, performs rescue breathing or CPR if trained to do so and facility allows it.		
6.	Stays with resident until help arrives.		

_____   _____
Date Reviewed   Instructor Signature

_____   _____
Date Performed   Instructor Signature

Seizures

		yes	no
1.	Notes time.		
2.	Lowers person to floor. Cradles and protects his head. Loosens clothing. Attempts to turn his head to one side.		
3.	Has someone call nurse immediately. Does not leave person unless must do so to get medical help.		
4.	Moves furniture away to prevent injury. If a pillow is nearby, places it under head.		
5.	Does not try to stop seizure or restrain person.		
6.	Does not force anything between person's teeth. Does not place hands in his mouth.		
7.	Does not give liquids or food.		

| 8. | When seizure is over, notes time. Checks breathing. | | |
| 9. | Reports length of seizure and observations to nurse. | | |

_____   _____
Date Reviewed   Instructor Signature

_____   _____
Date Performed   Instructor Signature

Admitting a resident

		yes	no
1.	Identifies self by name. Identifies resident and greets resident by name.		
2.	Washes hands.		
3.	Explains procedure to resident. Speaks clearly, slowly, and directly. Maintains face-to-face contact whenever possible. Encourages resident to assist if possible.		
4.	Provides for resident's privacy with a curtain, screen, or door.		
5.	If part of facility procedure, records resident's height, weight, and vital signs. Obtains a urine specimen if required. Completes paperwork and takes inventory of all personal items. Helps resident put personal items away. Labels each item if facility policy. Fills water pitcher if instructed.		
6.	Shows resident room and bathroom. Explains how to work bed controls and call light. Points out lights, telephone, and television and how to work them. Gives resident any information on menus, dining times, and activity schedules.		
7.	Introduces resident to his roommate, if there is one. Introduces other residents and staff.		
8.	Makes resident comfortable. Removes privacy measures.		

		yes	no
9.	Leaves call light within resident's reach.		
10.	Washes hands.		
11.	Is courteous and respectful at all times. Lets resident know when leaving. Asks if he needs anything else.		
12.	Documents procedure using facility guidelines.		

Date Reviewed _____ Instructor Signature _____

Date Performed _____ Instructor Signature _____

Measuring and recording weight of an ambulatory resident

		yes	no
1.	Identifies self by name. Identifies resident and greets resident by name.		
2.	Washes hands.		
3.	Explains procedure to resident. Speaks clearly, slowly, and directly. Maintains face-to-face contact whenever possible. Encourages resident to assist if possible.		
4.	Provides for resident's privacy with a curtain, screen, or door.		
5.	Starts with scale balanced at zero.		
6.	Helps resident remove shoes and step onto center of scale.		
7.	Weighs resident.		
8.	Helps resident off scale.		
9.	Records resident's weight.		
10.	Removes privacy measures.		
11.	Leaves call light within resident's reach.		
12.	Washes hands.		

		yes	no
13.	Is courteous and respectful at all times.		
14.	Reports any changes to nurse and documents procedure using facility guidelines.		

Date Reviewed _____ Instructor Signature _____

Date Performed _____ Instructor Signature _____

Measuring and recording weight of a bedridden resident

		yes	no
1.	Identifies self by name. Identifies resident and greets resident by name.		
2.	Washes hands.		
3.	Explains procedure to resident. Speaks clearly, slowly, and directly. Maintains face-to-face contact whenever possible. Encourages resident to assist if possible.		
4.	Provides for resident's privacy with a curtain, screen, or door.		
5.	Practices good body mechanics. Adjusts bed to a safe level, usually waist high. Locks bed wheels.		
6.	Starts with scale balanced at zero.		
7.	Examines sling, straps, chains, and/or pad for any damage.		
8.	Turns linen down so that it is off resident.		
9.	Turns resident to one side away from self or if flat pad scale is used, slides resident onto pad using a helper. If sling is used, removes sling from scale and places it underneath resident without wrinkling it.		
10.	With a sling, turns resident back to supine (back) position and straightens sling.		

Name: _____

11.	Attaches sling to scale or if using a flat pad scale, positions resident securely on pad.		
12.	Checks straps or other connectors, and raises sling or pad until resident is clear of bed. Secures resident.		
13.	Reads weight.		
14.	Lowers resident back down on bed. If using a sling, turns resident to both sides to remove sling. If using a pad scale, carefully slides resident back onto bed.		
15.	Records resident's weight.		
16.	Makes resident comfortable. Replaces bed linens.		
17.	Returns bed to low position if raised. Ensures resident's safety. Removes privacy measures.		
18.	Leaves call light within resident's reach.		
19.	Washes hands.		
20.	Is courteous and respectful at all times.		
21.	Reports any changes to nurse and documents procedure using facility guidelines.		

Date Reviewed _____ Instructor Signature _____

Date Performed _____ Instructor Signature _____

Measuring and recording height of an ambulatory resident

		yes	no
1.	Identifies self by name. Identifies resident and greets resident by name.		
2.	Washes hands.		
3.	Explains procedure to resident. Speaks clearly, slowly, and directly. Maintains face-to-face contact whenever possible. Encourages resident to assist if possible.		

4.	Provides for resident's privacy with a curtain, screen, or door.		
5.	Helps resident to step onto scale, facing away from scale.		
6.	Asks resident to stand straight. Helps as needed.		
7.	Pulls up measuring rod from back of scale. Gently lowers measuring rod until it rests flat on resident's head.		
8.	Determines resident's height.		
9.	Helps resident off scale before recording height.		
10.	Records height.		
11.	Removes privacy measures.		
12.	Leaves call light within resident's reach.		
13.	Washes hands.		
14.	Is courteous and respectful at all times.		
15.	Reports any changes to nurse and documents procedure using facility guidelines.		

Date Reviewed _____ Instructor Signature _____

Date Performed _____ Instructor Signature _____

Measuring and recording height of a bedridden resident

		yes	no
1.	Identifies self by name. Identifies resident and greets resident by name.		
2.	Washes hands.		
3.	Explains procedure to resident. Speaks clearly, slowly, and directly. Maintains face-to-face contact whenever possible. Encourages resident to assist if possible.		
4.	Provides for resident's privacy with a curtain, screen, or door.		

5.	Practices good body mechanics. Adjusts bed to a safe level, usually waist high. Locks bed wheels.		
6.	Turns linen down so it is off resident.		
7.	Positions resident lying straight in supine (back) position.		
8.	Using a pencil, makes a small mark on bottom sheet at top of resident's head.		
9.	Makes another pencil mark at bottom of resident's feet.		
10.	Using tape measure, measures area between pencil marks.		
11.	Records resident's height.		
12.	Makes resident comfortable and replaces bed linen.		
13.	Returns bed to low position if raised. Ensures resident's safety. Removes privacy measures.		
14.	Leaves call light within resident's reach.		
15.	Washes hands.		
16.	Is courteous and respectful at all times.		
17.	Reports any changes to nurse and documents procedure using facility guidelines.		

_____   _____
Date Reviewed   Instructor Signature

_____   _____
Date Performed   Instructor Signature

Measuring abdominal girth

		yes	no
1.	Identifies self by name. Identifies resident and greets resident by name.		
2.	Washes hands.		

3.	Explains procedure to resident. Speaks clearly, slowly, and directly. Maintains face-to-face contact whenever possible. Encourages resident to assist if possible.		
4.	Provides for resident's privacy with a curtain, screen, or door.		
5.	Practices good body mechanics. Adjusts bed to a safe level, usually waist high. Locks bed wheels.		
6.	Positions resident lying straight in supine (back) position.		
7.	Turns linen down and raises gown or top enough to expose only abdomen. Keeps all areas covered that do not need to be exposed.		
8.	Gently wraps measuring tape around resident's abdomen at level of navel.		
9.	Reads number where ends of tape meet.		
10.	Carefully removes tape measure. Records abdominal girth measurement.		
11.	Makes resident comfortable. Replaces clothing and bed linen.		
12.	Returns bed to low position if raised. Ensures resident's safety. Removes privacy measures.		
13.	Leaves call light within resident's reach.		
14.	Washes hands.		
15.	Is courteous and respectful at all times.		
16.	Reports any changes to nurse and documents procedure using facility guidelines.		

_____   _____
Date Reviewed   Instructor Signature

_____   _____
Date Performed   Instructor Signature

Transferring a resident

		yes	no
1.	Identifies self by name. Identifies resident and greets resident by name.		
2.	Washes hands.		
3.	Explains procedure to resident. Speaks clearly, slowly, and directly. Maintains face-to-face contact whenever possible. Encourages resident to assist if possible.		
4.	Provides for resident's privacy with a curtain, screen, or door.		
5.	Collects items to be moved onto cart, and takes them to new location.		
6.	Locks wheelchair or stretcher wheels. Helps resident into wheelchair or onto stretcher. Takes him or her to new area.		
7.	Introduces resident to new residents and staff.		
8.	Locks wheelchair or stretcher wheels. Transfers resident to new bed, if needed.		
9.	Unpacks all belongings. Helps resident to put personal items away.		
10.	Makes resident comfortable.		
11.	Leaves call light within resident's reach.		
12.	Washes hands.		
13.	Is courteous and respectful at all times.		
14.	Reports any changes to nurse and documents procedure using facility guidelines.		

_____ _____
Date Reviewed   Instructor Signature

_____ _____
Date Performed   Instructor Signature

Discharging a resident

		yes	no
1.	Identifies self by name. Identifies resident and greets resident by name.		
2.	Washes hands.		
3.	Explains procedure to resident. Speaks clearly, slowly, and directly. Maintains face-to-face contact whenever possible. Encourages resident to assist if possible.		
4.	Provides for resident's privacy with a curtain, screen, or door.		
5.	Compares inventory list to items being packed. Asks resident to sign if all items are there.		
6.	Carefully puts items to be taken onto cart and transports items to pick-up area.		
7.	Helps resident dress in clothing of his choice.		
8.	Helps resident safely into wheelchair or onto stretcher.		
9.	Helps resident to say goodbye to other residents and staff.		
10.	Takes resident to pick-up area. Helps him into vehicle. Transfers personal items into vehicle.		
11.	Says goodbye to resident.		
12.	Washes hands.		
13.	Documents procedure using facility guidelines.		

_____ _____
Date Reviewed   Instructor Signature

_____ _____
Date Performed   Instructor Signature

Making a closed bed

		yes	no
1.	Washes hands.		
2.	Gathers linen. Transports linen correctly.		

3.	If resident is in room, identifies self by name. Identifies resident and greets resident by name.		
4.	Explains procedure to resident. Speaks clearly, slowly, and directly. Maintains face-to-face contact whenever possible.		
5.	Places clean linen on clean surface within reach.		
6.	Adjusts bed to safe working level. Puts bed in flattest position.		
7.	Applies gloves.		
8.	Loosens soiled linen and rolls soiled linen (soiled side inside) from head to foot of bed. Places it in a hamper or linen bag.		
9.	Removes and disposes of gloves properly. Washes hands.		
10.	Remakes bed. Places mattress pad (if used) on bed, attaching elastic at corners as necessary.		
11.	Places bottom sheet on bed without shaking linen. If using a flat sheet with seams, places sheet with crease in center of mattress with seams on both ends down. If using a fitted bottom sheet, places right-side up and tightly pulls over all four corners of bed.		
12.	Makes hospital corners to keep bottom sheet wrinkle-free.		
13.	Puts on waterproof bed protector and then draw sheet, if used. Places them in center of bed on bottom sheet. Smoothes and tightly tucks bottom sheet and draw sheet together under sides of bed. Moves from head of bed to foot of bed.		
14.	Places top sheet over bed and centers it with seam up.		
15.	Places blanket over bed and centers it.		
16.	Places bedspread over bed and centers it.		

17.	Tucks top sheet, blanket, and bedspread under foot of bed and makes hospital corners.		
18.	Folds down top sheet to make a cuff of about six inches over blanket and bedspread.		
19.	Takes a pillow, and with one hand, grasps clean pillowcase at closed end. Turns it inside out over arm. Using hand that has pillowcase over it, grasps center of end of pillow. Pulls pillowcase over it with free hand. Places pillows at head of bed with open end away from door. Makes sure zippers or tags are inside.		
20.	Returns bed to low position if raised.		
21.	Disposes of soiled linen in proper container.		
22.	Leaves call light within resident's reach.		
23.	Washes hands.		
24.	Documents procedure using facility guidelines.		

_____   _____
Date Reviewed   Instructor Signature

_____   _____
Date Performed   Instructor Signature

Making an open bed		yes	no
1.	Washes hands.		
2.	Makes a closed bed.		
3.	Stands at head of bed. Grasps top sheet, blanket, and bedspread and folds them down to foot of bed. Then brings them back up bed to form a large cuff.		
4.	Brings cuff on top linens to a point where it is one hand-width above linen underneath.		
5.	Makes sure all linen is wrinkle-free.		
6.	Washes hands.		

7.	Documents procedure using facility guidelines.		

_____   _____
Date Reviewed   Instructor Signature

_____   _____
Date Performed   Instructor Signature

Making an occupied bed

		yes	no
1.	Washes hands.		
2.	Gathers linen. Transports linen correctly.		
3.	Identifies self by name. Identifies resident and greets resident by name.		
4.	Explains procedure to resident. Speaks clearly, slowly, and directly. Maintains face-to-face contact whenever possible. Encourages resident to assist if possible.		
5.	Places clean linen within reach.		
6.	Provides for resident's privacy with a curtain, screen, or door and avoids trauma or pain to resident throughout procedure.		
7.	Puts on gloves.		
8.	Covers resident and loosens top linens.		
9.	Unfolds bath blanket over top sheet and removes top sheet, keeping resident covered at all times.		
10.	Practices good body mechanics. Adjusts bed to safe working level. Lowers head of bed. Locks bed wheels.		
11.	Makes bed one side at a time. Raises side rail on far side of bed. Goes to other side of bed and lowers side rail. Helps resident to turn onto his side.		
12.	Loosens bottom soiled linen on working side.		

13.	Rolls bottom soiled linen toward resident and center of bed, soiled side inside. Tucks it snugly against resident's back.		
14.	Places mattress pad on bed, attaching elastic at corners on working side.		
15.	Places clean bottom linen or fitted bottom sheet with center crease centered. If flat sheet is used, tucks in at top and on working side. Makes hospital corners. If fitted sheet is used, tightly pulls two fitted corners on working side.		
16.	Smoothes bottom sheet out toward resident. Rolls extra material toward resident and tucks it under resident's body.		
17.	If using a waterproof bed protector, unfolds it and centers it on bed. Smoothes it out toward resident.		
18.	If using a draw sheet, places it on bed. Tucks in on working side, smoothes, and tucks as with other bedding.		
19.	Raises near side rail. Goes to other side of bed and lowers side rail. Helps resident roll or turn onto clean bottom sheet, explaining that he will be moving over a roll of linen.		
20.	Loosens soiled linen. Rolls linen from head to foot of bed, avoiding contact with skin or clothes. Does not shake soiled linen. Places it in a hamper or linen bag.		

21.	Pulls clean linen through as quickly as possible. Starts with mattress pad and wraps around corners. Pulls and tucks in clean bottom linen. Pulls and tucks in waterproof bed protector and draw sheet, if used. Makes hospital corners with bottom sheet. Finishes with bottom sheet free of wrinkles.		
22.	Places resident on his back. Keeps resident covered and comfortable, with a pillow under his head.		
23.	Unfolds top sheet. Places it over resident and centers it. Asks resident to hold top sheet and slips bath blanket out from underneath. Puts in hamper/bag.		
24.	Places blanket over top sheet and centers it. Places bedspread over blanket and centers it. Tucks top sheet, blanket and bedspread under foot of bed and makes hospital corners on each side. Loosens top linens over resident's feet.		
25.	At top of bed, folds down top sheet to make a cuff of about six inches over blanket and bedspread.		
26.	Gently holds and lifts resident's head and removes pillow. Does not hold it near face.		
27.	Removes soiled pillowcase by turning it inside out. Places it in hamper/bag.		
28.	With one hand, grasps clean pillowcase at closed end. Turns it inside out over arm. Using hand that has pillowcase over it, grasps center of end of pillow. Pulls pillowcase over it with free hand. Places pillows gently under resident's head with open end away from door. Makes sure zippers or tags are inside.		

29.	Makes sure bed is wrinkle-free. Makes resident comfortable.		
30.	Returns bed to low position. Ensures resident's safety. Returns side rails to ordered position. Removes privacy measures.		
31.	Leaves call light within resident's reach.		
32.	Disposes of soiled linen in proper container.		
33.	Removes and disposes of gloves properly.		
34.	Washes hands.		
35.	Is courteous and respectful at all times.		
36.	Reports any changes to nurse and documents procedure using facility guidelines.		

Date Reviewed _____ Instructor Signature _____

Date Performed _____ Instructor Signature _____

Making a surgical bed

		yes	no
1.	Washes hands.		
2.	Gathers linen. Transports linen correctly.		
3.	Places clean linen within reach.		
4.	Adjusts bed to safe working level. Locks bed wheels.		
5.	Applies gloves.		
6.	Removes all soiled linen, rolling it (soiled side inside) from head to foot of bed. Avoids contact with skin or clothes. Places it in hamper or linen bag.		
7.	Removes and disposes of gloves properly.		
8.	Washes hands.		
9.	Makes a closed bed. Does not tuck top linens under mattress.		

Name: _____

10.	Folds top linens down from head of bed and up from foot of bed.		
11.	Forms triangle with linen. Fanfolds linen triangle into pleated layers and positions opposite stretcher side of bed. After fanfolding, forms a tiny tip with end of linen triangle.		
12.	Puts on clean pillowcases. Places clean pillows on a clean surface off bed.		
13.	Leaves bed in highest position. Leaves both side rails down.		
14.	Moves all furniture to make room for stretcher.		
15.	Does not place call light on bed.		
16.	Disposes of soiled linen in proper container.		
17.	Washes hands.		
18.	Documents procedure using facility guidelines.		

_____   _____
Date Reviewed   Instructor Signature

_____   _____
Date Performed   Instructor Signature

Locking arms with a resident and raising head and shoulders

		yes	no
1.	Identifies self by name. Identifies resident and greets resident by name.		
2.	Washes hands.		
3.	Explains procedure to resident. Speaks clearly, slowly, and directly. Maintains face-to-face contact whenever possible. Encourages resident to assist if possible.		
4.	Provides for resident's privacy with a curtain, screen, or door.		
5.	Practices good body mechanics. Adjusts bed to a safe level. Locks bed wheels.		

6.	Places pillow at head of bed against headboard.		
7.	Lowers side rail on side nearest self.		
8.	Stands at side of bed and faces head of bed.		
9.	Gently slides one hand under resident's closest shoulder.		
10.	Gently slides other hand under resident's upper back.		
11.	On signal, slowly raises resident's head and shoulders. Gives necessary care.		
12.	Replaces pillow under resident's head.		
13.	Makes resident comfortable.		
14.	Returns bed to low position if raised. Ensures resident's safety. Returns side rails to ordered position. Removes privacy measures.		
15.	Leaves call light within resident's reach.		
16.	Washes hands.		
17.	Is courteous and respectful at all times.		
18.	Reports any changes to nurse and documents procedure using facility guidelines.		

_____   _____
Date Reviewed   Instructor Signature

_____   _____
Date Performed   Instructor Signature

Assisting a resident to move up in bed

		yes	no
1.	Identifies self by name. Identifies resident and greets resident by name.		
2.	Washes hands.		

3.	Explains procedure to resident. Speaks clearly, slowly, and directly. Maintains face-to-face contact whenever possible. Encourages resident to assist if possible.		
4.	Provides for resident's privacy with a curtain, screen, or door.		
5.	Practices good body mechanics. Adjusts bed to a safe level. Locks bed wheels.		
6.	Lowers head of bed. Moves pillow to head of bed.		
7.	Lowers side rail on side nearest self.		
8.	Stands by bed with feet apart, facing resident.		
9.	Places one arm under resident's shoulder blades. Places other arm under resident's thighs.		
10.	Asks resident to bend knees, brace feet on mattress, and push feet on count of three.		
11.	On signal, shifts body weight to move resident while resident pushes with her feet.		
12.	Replaces pillow under resident's head.		
13.	Makes resident comfortable.		
14.	Returns bed to low position if raised. Ensures resident's safety. Returns side rails to ordered position. Removes privacy measures.		
15.	Leaves call light within resident's reach.		
16.	Washes hands.		
17.	Is courteous and respectful at all times.		
18.	Reports any changes to nurse and documents procedure using facility guidelines.		

_____   _____
Date Reviewed   Instructor Signature

_____   _____
Date Performed   Instructor Signature

Assisting a resident to move up in bed with assistance (using draw sheet)

		yes	no
1.	Identifies self by name. Identifies resident and greets resident by name.		
2.	Washes hands.		
3.	Explains procedure to resident. Speaks clearly, slowly, and directly. Maintains face-to-face contact whenever possible. Encourages resident to assist if possible.		
4.	Provides for resident's privacy with a curtain, screen, or door.		
5.	Adjusts bed to a safe level, usually waist high. Locks bed wheels.		
6.	Lowers head of bed. Moves pillow to head of bed.		
7.	Lowers side rail on side nearest self.		
8.	Stands on opposite side of bed from helper. Turns slightly toward head of bed. Stands with feet about 12 inches apart and knees bent.		
9.	Rolls draw sheet up to resident's side. Grasps sheet with palms up.		
10.	Shifts weight to back foot and has helper do same. On signal, shifts weight to forward feet. Slides resident toward head of bed.		
11.	Replaces pillow under resident's head.		
12.	Makes resident comfortable. Unrolls draw sheet. Leaves it in place for next repositioning.		
13.	Returns bed to low position if raised. Ensures resident's safety. Returns side rails to ordered position. Removes privacy measures.		

14.	Leaves call light within resident's reach.		
15.	Washes hands.		
16.	Is courteous and respectful at all times.		
17.	Reports any changes to nurse and documents procedure using facility guidelines.		

_____ _____
Date Reviewed   Instructor Signature

_____ _____
Date Performed   Instructor Signature

Moving a resident to the side of the bed

		yes	no
1.	Identifies self by name. Identifies resident and greets resident by name.		
2.	Washes hands.		
3.	Explains procedure to resident. Speaks clearly, slowly, and directly. Maintains face-to-face contact whenever possible. Encourages resident to assist if possible.		
4.	Provides for resident's privacy with a curtain, screen, or door.		
5.	Practices good body mechanics. Adjusts bed to a safe level. Locks bed wheels.		
6.	Lowers head of bed. Moves pillow to head of bed.		
7.	Stands on one side of bed. Lowers side rail on near side.		
8.	Gently slides hands under resident's head and shoulders and moves toward self. Gently slides hands under resident's midsection and moves toward self. Gently slides hands under resident's hips and legs and moves toward self.		
9.	Makes resident comfortable. Repositions pillow under head.		

10.	Returns bed to low position if raised. Ensures resident's safety. Returns side rails to ordered position. Removes privacy measures.		
11.	Leaves call light within resident's reach.		
12.	Washes hands.		
13.	Is courteous and respectful at all times.		
14.	Reports any changes to nurse and documents procedure using facility guidelines.		

_____ _____
Date Reviewed   Instructor Signature

_____ _____
Date Performed   Instructor Signature

Moving a resident to the side of the bed with assistance (using draw sheet)

		yes	no
1.	Identifies self by name. Identifies resident and greets resident by name.		
2.	Washes hands.		
3.	Explains procedure to resident. Speaks clearly, slowly, and directly. Maintains face-to-face contact whenever possible. Encourages resident to assist if possible.		
4.	Provides for resident's privacy with a curtain, screen, or door.		
5.	Practices good body mechanics. Adjusts bed to a safe level, usually waist high. Locks bed wheels.		
6.	Lowers head of bed. Moves pillow to head of bed.		
7.	Stands on opposite side of bed from helper. Lowers both side rails. Stands up straight facing side of bed with feet about 12 inches apart.		

Name: _____

8.	Rolls draw sheet up to resident's side. Has helper do same. Grasps sheet with palms up at resident's shoulders and hips and has helper do same.		
9.	On signal, slides resident toward side of bed.		
10.	Makes resident comfortable. Unrolls draw sheet. Leaves it in place for next repositioning. Repositions pillow under head.		
11.	Returns bed to low position if raised. Ensures resident's safety. Returns side rails to ordered position. Removes privacy measures.		
12.	Leaves call light within resident's reach.		
13.	Washes hands.		
14.	Is courteous and respectful at all times.		
15.	Reports any changes to nurse and documents procedure using facility guidelines.		

_____ _____
Date Reviewed   Instructor Signature

_____ _____
Date Performed   Instructor Signature

Turning a resident away from you

		yes	no
1.	Identifies self by name. Identifies resident and greets resident by name.		
2.	Washes hands.		
3.	Explains procedure to resident. Speaks clearly, slowly, and directly. Maintains face-to-face contact whenever possible. Encourages resident to assist if possible.		
4.	Provides for resident's privacy with a curtain, screen, or door.		
5.	Practices good body mechanics. Adjusts bed to a safe level. Locks bed wheels.		

6.	Lowers head of bed.		
7.	Stands on side of bed opposite to where person will be turned with far side rail raised.		
8.	Lowers near side rail.		
9.	Moves resident to side of bed nearest self.		
10.	Crosses resident's arm over chest. Moves arm out of way on side toward which resident is being turned. Crosses leg nearest self over far leg.		
11.	Stands with feet about 12 inches apart and bends knees.		
12.	Places one hand on resident's shoulder. Places other hand on resident's nearest hip.		
13.	Gently pushes resident toward other side of bed. Shifts weight from back leg to front leg. Makes sure resident's face is not covered by pillow.		
14.	Positions resident properly in good alignment, including:		
a.	head supported by pillow		
b.	shoulder adjusted so resident is not lying on arm		
c.	top arm supported by pillow		
d.	back supported by supportive device		
e.	hips properly aligned		
f.	top knee flexed		
g.	supportive device between legs with top knee flexed; knee and ankle supported		
15.	Covers resident with top linens and straightens. Makes resident comfortable.		
16.	Returns bed to low position if raised. Ensures resident's safety. Returns side rails to ordered position. Removes privacy measures.		

Name: _____

17.	Leaves call light within resident's reach.		
18.	Washes hands.		
19.	Is courteous and respectful at all times.		
20.	Reports any changes to nurse and documents procedure using facility guidelines.		

_____   _____
Date Reviewed   Instructor Signature

_____   _____
Date Performed   Instructor Signature

Turning a resident toward you

		yes	no
1.	Identifies self by name. Identifies resident and greets resident by name.		
2.	Washes hands.		
3.	Explains procedure to resident. Speaks clearly, slowly, and directly. Maintains face-to-face contact whenever possible. Encourages resident to assist if possible.		
4.	Provides for resident's privacy with a curtain, screen, or door.		
5.	Practices good body mechanics. Adjusts bed to a safe level. Locks bed wheels.		
6.	Lowers head of bed.		
7.	Stands on side of bed opposite to where person will be turned with far side rail raised.		
8.	Lowers side rail nearest self.		
9.	Moves resident to side of bed nearest self. Puts side rail up and goes to opposite side of bed. Lowers side rail.		
10.	Crosses resident's arm over chest. Moves arm out of way on side toward which resident is being turned. Crosses far leg over near leg.		
11.	Stands with feet about 12 inches apart and bends knees.		
12.	Places one hand on resident's far shoulder. Places other hand on resident's far hip.		
13.	While supporting body, gently rolls resident toward self. Makes sure resident's face is not covered by pillow.		
14.	Positions resident properly in good alignment, including:		
a.	head supported by pillow		
b.	shoulder adjusted so resident is not lying on arm		
c.	top arm supported by pillow		
d.	back supported by supportive device		
e.	hips properly aligned		
f.	top knee flexed		
g.	supportive device between legs with top knee flexed; knee and ankle supported		
15.	Covers resident with top linens and straightens. Makes resident comfortable.		
16.	Returns bed to low position if raised. Ensures resident's safety. Returns side rails to ordered position. Removes privacy measures.		
17.	Leaves call light within resident's reach.		
18.	Washes hands.		
19.	Is courteous and respectful at all times.		
20.	Reports any changes to nurse and documents procedure using facility guidelines.		

_____   _____
Date Reviewed   Instructor Signature

_____   _____
Date Performed   Instructor Signature

Logrolling a resident with assistance

		yes	no
1.	Identifies self by name. Identifies resident. Greets resident by name.		
2.	Washes hands.		
3.	Explains procedure to resident. Speaks clearly, slowly, and directly. Maintains face-to-face contact whenever possible. Encourages resident to assist if possible.		
4.	Provides for resident's privacy with a curtain, screen, or door.		
5.	Practices good body mechanics. Adjusts bed to a safe level. Locks bed wheels.		
6.	Lowers head of bed.		
7.	Stands on same side of bed as helper. Lowers side rail on side nearest self.		
8.	Places a pillow under resident's head to support neck during move.		
9.	Places resident's arms across chest. Places a pillow between knees.		
10.	Stands with feet about 12 inches apart. Bends knees.		
11.	Grasps draw sheet on far side.		
12.	On signal, gently rolls resident toward self. Turns resident as a unit.		
13.	Repositions resident comfortably in good alignment. Places pillow under head. Covers resident with top linens and straightens.		
14.	Returns bed to low position if raised. Ensures resident's safety. Returns side rails to ordered position. Removes privacy measures.		
15.	Leaves call light within resident's reach.		
16.	Washes hands.		
17.	Is courteous and respectful at all times.		
18.	Reports any changes to nurse and documents procedure using facility guidelines.		

_____   _____
Date Reviewed   Instructor Signature

_____   _____
Date Performed   Instructor Signature

Assisting a resident to sit up on side of bed: dangling

		yes	no
1.	Identifies self by name. Identifies resident and greets resident by name.		
2.	Washes hands.		
3.	Explains procedure to resident. Speaks clearly, slowly, and directly. Maintains face-to-face contact whenever possible. Encourages resident to assist if possible.		
4.	Provides for resident's privacy with a curtain, screen, or door.		
5.	Practices good body mechanics. Adjusts bed to lowest safe working level. Locks bed wheels.		
6.	Raises head of bed to sitting position. Folds linen to foot of bed. Lowers side rail on side nearest self.		
7.	Stands at side of bed with feet about 12 inches apart. Helps resident slowly move toward near side of bed.		
8.	Places one arm under resident's shoulder blades. Places other arm under resident's thighs.		

Name: _____

9.	On signal, gently and slowly turns resident into sitting position with legs dangling over side of bed.		
10.	Asks resident to sit up straight and push both fists into edge of mattress. Assists resident to put on robe.		
11.	Has resident dangle as long as ordered. Places pillow or other supporting device behind resident's back during dangle. Stays with resident at all times. Checks for dizziness. If resident feels dizzy or faint, helps her lie down again and makes sure she is secure. Tells nurse at once.		
12.	Takes vital signs as ordered.		
13.	Gently assists resident back into bed. Places one arm around resident's shoulders. Places other arm under resident's knees. Slowly swings resident's legs onto bed.		
14.	Makes resident comfortable. Covers resident with top linens and straightens. Replaces pillow under resident's head.		
15.	Returns bed to low position if raised. Ensures resident's safety. Returns side rails to ordered position. Removes privacy measures.		
16.	Leaves call light within resident's reach.		
17.	Washes hands.		
18.	Is courteous and respectful at all times.		
19.	Reports any changes to nurse and documents procedure using facility guidelines.		

_____   _____
Date Reviewed   Instructor Signature

_____   _____
Date Performed   Instructor Signature

Applying a transfer belt

		yes	no
1.	Identifies self by name. Identifies resident and greets resident by name.		
2.	Washes hands.		
3.	Explains procedure to resident. Speaks clearly, slowly, and directly. Maintains face-to-face contact whenever possible. Encourages resident to assist if possible.		
4.	Provides for resident's privacy with a curtain, screen, or door.		
5.	Practices good body mechanics. Adjusts bed to low, flat position. Locks bed wheels.		
6.	Supporting back and hips, assists resident to a sitting position with feet flat on floor.		
7.	Puts on and properly fastens non-skid footwear on resident.		
8.	Places belt over resident's clothing below rib cage and above waist. Does not put it over bare skin.		
9.	Tightens buckle until snug. Leaves enough room to insert three fingers into belt.		
10.	Checks to make sure that resident's breasts are not caught under belt.		
11.	Positions buckle slightly off-center in front or back for comfort.		

_____   _____
Date Reviewed   Instructor Signature

_____   _____
Date Performed   Instructor Signature

Transferring a resident from bed to a chair or wheelchair

		yes	no
1.	Identifies self by name. Identifies resident and greets resident by name.		

2.	Washes hands.		
3.	Explains procedure to resident. Speaks clearly, slowly, and directly. Maintains face-to-face contact whenever possible. Encourages resident to assist if possible.		
4.	Provides for resident's privacy with a curtain, screen, or door.		
5.	Practices good body mechanics.		
6.	Removes wheelchair footrests close to bed.		
7.	Places wheelchair near head of bed with arm of wheelchair almost touching bed. Places wheelchair on resident's stronger, or unaffected, side. Lowers side rail on side nearest self.		
8.	Locks wheelchair wheels.		
9.	Raises head of bed. Adjusts bed level. Locks bed wheels.		
10.	Assists resident to sitting position with feet flat on floor. Lets resident sit for a few minutes.		
11.	Puts non-skid footwear on resident and securely fastens.		
13.	With transfer (gait) belt:		
	a. Stands in front of resident.		
	b. Stands with feet about 12 inches apart. Bends knees. Keeps back straight.		
	c. Places belt below rib cage and above waist. Does not put it over bare skin. Grasps belt securely on both sides.		
	Without transfer belt:		
	a. Stands in front of resident.		
	b. Stands with feet about 12 inches apart. Bends knees. Keeps back straight.		
	c. Places arms around resident's torso under arms, but not in armpits.		
13.	Provides instructions to allow resident to help with transfer.		

14.	With legs, braces resident's lower legs to prevent slipping.		
15.	Alerts resident, then slowly helps resident to stand.		
16.	Helps resident to pivot to front of wheelchair with back of resident's legs against wheelchair.		
17.	Asks resident to put hands on wheelchair armrests if able.		
18.	Gently lowers resident into wheelchair.		
19	Repositions resident with hips touching back of wheelchair. Removes transfer belt, if used.		
20.	Attaches footrests. Places resident's feet on footrests.		
21.	Makes resident comfortable.		
22.	Removes privacy measures.		
23.	Leaves call light within resident's reach.		
24.	Washes hands.		
25.	Is courteous and respectful at all times.		
26.	Reports any changes in resident to nurse. Documents procedure using facility guidelines.		
	To transfer back to bed from wheelchair, follows these steps:		
1.	Performs steps 1 through 8 above.		
2.	Adjusts bed level to a low position. Locks bed wheels.		
3.	Avoids trauma or pain to resident throughout procedure.		
4.	Performs steps 13 through 16 above. Allows resident to stand until he feels stable enough to move toward bed.		
5.	Helps resident to pivot to bed with back of resident's legs against bed.		
6.	Makes resident comfortable. Removes transfer belt, if used.		

Name: _____

7.	Returns bed to low position if raised. Ensures resident's safety. Returns side rails to ordered position. Removes privacy measures.		
8.	Leaves call light within resident's reach.		
9.	Washes hands.		
10.	Is courteous and respectful at all times.		
11.	Reports any changes to nurse and documents procedure using facility guidelines.		

_____ _____
Date Reviewed   Instructor Signature

_____ _____
Date Performed   Instructor Signature

Transferring a resident from bed to stretcher with assistance

		yes	no
1.	Identifies self by name. Identifies resident and greets resident by name.		
2.	Washes hands.		
3.	Explains procedure to resident. Speaks clearly, slowly, and directly. Maintains face-to-face contact whenever possible. Encourages resident to assist if possible.		
4.	Provides for resident's privacy with a curtain, screen, or door.		
5.	Practices good body mechanics. Lowers head of bed so that it is flat. Locks bed wheels.		
6.	Folds linens to foot of bed. Covers resident with bath blanket.		
7.	Lowers side rail on side to which resident will be moved.		
8.	Moves resident to side of bed.		

9.	Places stretcher solidly against bed. Locks stretcher wheels. Moves stretcher safety belts out of way.		
10.	Two workers are on side of bed opposite stretcher. Two more workers are on outside of stretcher.		
11.	Each worker rolls up sides of draw sheet and prepares to move resident, protecting resident's arms and legs during transfer.		
12.	On signal, workers lift and move resident to stretcher. All move at once. Resident is centered on stretcher.		
13.	Raises head of stretcher or places pillow under resident's head if allowed.		
14.	Places safety straps across resident. Raises side rails on stretcher.		
15.	Unlocks stretcher's wheels. Takes resident to appropriate site. Stays with resident until another team member takes over.		
16.	Washes hands.		
17.	Is courteous and respectful at all times.		
18.	Reports any changes to nurse and documents procedure using facility guidelines.		

_____ _____
Date Reviewed   Instructor Signature

_____ _____
Date Performed   Instructor Signature

Transferring a resident using a mechanical lift with assistance

		yes	no
1.	Identifies self by name. Identifies resident and greets resident by name.		
2.	Washes hands.		

3.	Explains procedure to resident. Speaks clearly, slowly, and directly. Maintains face-to-face contact whenever possible. Encourages resident to assist if possible.		
4.	Provides for resident's privacy with a curtain, screen, or door.		
5.	Practices good body mechanics. Lowers bed to proper position for move. Locks bed wheels.		
6.	Removes wheelchair footrests close to bed.		
7.	Positions wheelchair next to bed. Lowers side rail on near side. Locks wheelchair brakes.		
8.	Helps resident turn to one side of bed. Pads sling where neck will rest with a washcloth. Positions sling under resident, with edge next to resident's back. Fanfolds. Makes bottom of sling even with resident's knees. Helps resident roll to his opposite side. Spreads out fanfolded edge of sling, then rolls back to middle of bed.		
9.	Rolls mechanical lift to bedside. Makes sure base is opened to its widest point. Pushes base of lift under bed. Locks lift wheels.		
10.	Places overhead bar directly over resident.		
11.	With resident lying on her back, attaches one set of straps to each side of sling. Attaches one set of straps to overhead bar.		
12.	Following manufacturer's instructions, raises resident two inches above bed. Pauses a moment for resident to gain balance.		
13.	Slowly lowers resident into chair or wheelchair. Pushes down gently on resident's knees to help resident into sitting position.		

14.	Undoes straps from overhead bar. Leaves sling in place for transfer back to bed.		
15.	Makes sure resident is seated comfortably and correctly in chair or wheelchair. Puts non-skid footwear on resident and fastens. Replaces footrests. Covers resident with a lap cover or robe if he requests it.		
16.	Removes privacy measures.		
17.	Leaves call light within resident's reach.		
18.	Washes hands.		
19.	Is courteous and respectful at all times.		
20.	Reports any changes to nurse and documents procedure using facility guidelines.		

_____   _____
Date Reviewed   Instructor Signature

_____   _____
Date Performed   Instructor Signature

Transferring a resident onto and off a toilet

		yes	no
1.	Identifies self by name. Identifies resident and greets resident by name.		
2.	Washes hands.		
3.	Explains procedure to resident. Speaks clearly, slowly, and directly. Maintains face-to-face contact whenever possible. Encourages resident to assist if possible.		
4.	Provides for resident's privacy with a curtain, screen, or door.		
5.	Practices good body mechanics.		
6.	Positions wheelchair at a right angle to toilet to face hand bar/wall rail. Places wheelchair on resident's stronger side, if possible.		

Name: _____

7.	Removes wheelchair footrests. Locks wheels. Puts on and properly fastens non-skid footwear on resident.		
8.	Applies a transfer belt around resident's waist. Grasps belt. Puts one hand toward resident's back and one toward resident's front.		
9.	Asks resident to push against armrests of wheelchair and stand, reaching for and grasping hand bar with his stronger arm.		
10.	Asks resident to pivot feet and back up so that he can feel front of toilet with back of his legs.		
11.	Helps resident to pull down underwear and pants.		
12.	Helps resident to slowly sit down onto toilet. Removes transfer belt. Allows privacy unless resident cannot be left alone. Asks resident to pull on emergency cord if he needs help. Closes bathroom door. Stays near door until resident is finished.		
13.	When resident is finished, applies gloves. Assists with perineal care as necessary. Reapplies transfer belt if removed. Asks him to stand and reach for hand bar.		
14.	Uses toilet tissue or damp cloth to clean resident. Makes sure he is clean and dry before pulling up clothing. Removes and disposes of gloves.		
15.	Pulls up resident's clothing. Helps resident to sink to wash hands. Washes hands.		
16.	Helps resident back into wheelchair. Makes sure resident is seated comfortably and correctly in chair or wheelchair. Replaces footrests.		

17.	Helps resident to leave bathroom.		
18.	Leaves call light within resident's reach.		
19.	Washes hands.		
20.	Is courteous and respectful at all times.		
21.	Reports any changes to nurse and documents procedure using facility guidelines.		

_____   _____
Date Reviewed   Instructor Signature

_____   _____
Date Performed   Instructor Signature

Transferring a resident into a car

		yes	no
1.	Identifies self by name. Identifies resident and greets resident by name.		
2.	Washes hands.		
3.	Explains procedure to resident. Speaks clearly, slowly, and directly. Maintains face-to-face contact whenever possible. Encourages resident to assist if possible.		
4.	Practices good body mechanics.		
5.	Places wheelchair close to car at a 45-degree angle. Opens door on resident's stronger side.		
6.	Locks wheelchair.		
7.	Asks resident to push against arm rests of wheelchair and stand.		
8.	Asks resident to stand, grasp car or dashboard, and pivot his foot so side of car seat touches back of legs.		
9.	Asks resident to sit in seat and lift one leg, then the other, into vehicle.		
10.	Carefully positions resident comfortably in car. Helps secure seat belt.		

11.	Sees that door can be safely shut. Shuts door.		
12.	Returns wheelchair to appropriate place for cleaning.		
13.	Washes hands.		
14.	Documents procedure using facility guidelines.		

_____ _____
Date Reviewed   Instructor Signature

_____ _____
Date Performed   Instructor Signature

Assisting a resident to ambulate

		yes	no
1.	Identifies self by name. Identifies resident and greets resident by name.		
2.	Washes hands.		
3.	Explains procedure to resident. Speaks clearly, slowly, and directly. Maintains face-to-face contact whenever possible. Encourages resident to assist if possible.		
4.	Provides for resident's privacy with a curtain, screen, or door.		
5.	Helps resident move to a dangling position.		
6.	Practices good body mechanics. Adjusts bed to a low position so that resident's feet are flat on floor. Locks bed wheels.		
7.	Puts on and properly fastens non-skid footwear for resident.		
8.	Stands in front of and faces resident.		
9.	Braces resident's lower extremities. Bends knees. If resident has a weak knee, braces his knee against your knee.		
10.	**With transfer (gait) belt**: Places belt around resident's waist. Grasps belt while assisting resident to stand.		
	Without transfer belt: Places arms around resident's torso under arms, but not in armpits, while assisting resident to stand.		
11.	**With transfer belt**: Walks slightly behind and to one side of resident for full distance, while holding onto transfer belt. If resident has a weaker side, stands on weaker side. Asks resident to look forward during ambulation. If resident becomes dizzy or faint, helps him to a nearby seat and calls nurse for help.		
	Without transfer belt: Walks slightly behind and to one side of resident for full distance. Supports resident's back with arm. Asks resident to look forward during ambulation. If resident becomes dizzy or faint, helps him to a nearby seat and calls nurse for help.		
12.	After ambulation, makes resident comfortable. Removes transfer belt, if used.		
13.	Returns bed to low position if raised. Ensures resident's safety. Removes privacy measures.		
14.	Leaves call light within resident's reach.		
15.	Washes hands.		
16.	Is courteous and respectful at all times.		
17.	Reports any changes to nurse and documents procedure using facility guidelines.		

_____ _____
Date Reviewed   Instructor Signature

_____ _____
Date Performed   Instructor Signature

Giving a complete bed bath

		yes	no
1.	Identifies self by name. Identifies resident and greets resident by name.		
2.	Washes hands.		
3.	Explains procedure to resident. Speaks clearly, slowly, and directly. Maintains face-to-face contact whenever possible. Encourages resident to assist if possible.		
4.	Provides for resident's privacy with a curtain, screen, or door. Makes sure room is at a comfortable temperature and there are no drafts.		
5.	Practices good body mechanics. Adjusts bed to safe working level. Locks bed wheels.		
6.	Adjusts position of side rails to ensure resident safety at all times.		
7.	Places a bath blanket or towel over resident. Asks him to hold onto it and removes or folds back top bedding. Keeps resident covered with bath blanket.		
8.	Fills basin with warm water. Tests water temperature with thermometer or wrist and ensures it is safe. Has resident check water temperature. Adjusts if necessary. Changes water when it becomes too cool, soapy, or dirty.		
9.	If resident has open wounds, puts on gloves. Asks resident to participate in washing. Helps him do this whenever needed.		
10.	Uncovers only one part of body at a time. Places a towel under body part being washed.		
11.	Washes, rinses, and dries one part of body at a time. Starts at head. Works down, and completes front first. Folds washcloth over hand like a mitt and holds it in place with thumb.		
	Eyes, Face, Ears, Neck: Washes face with wet washcloth (no soap). Begins with far eye. Washes inner aspect to outer aspect. Uses a different area of washcloth for each eye. Washes face from middle outward. Uses firm but gentle strokes. Washes ears and behind ears and neck. Rinses and pats dry with blotting motion.		
	Arms and Axillae: Removes resident's top clothing. Covers him with bath blanket or towel. With a soapy washcloth, washes upper arm and underarm. Uses long strokes from shoulder to elbow. Rinses and pats dry. Washes elbow. Washes, rinses, and dries from elbow down to wrist.		
	Hands: Washes hand in basin. Cleans under nails with orangewood stick or nail brush. Rinses and pats dry. Makes sure to dry between fingers. Gives nail care if assigned. Repeats for other arm. Puts lotion on resident's elbows and hands if ordered.		
	Chest: Places towel across resident's chest. Pulls bath blanket down to waist. Lifts towel only enough to wash chest. Rinses it and pats dry. For a female resident, washes, rinses, and dries breasts and under breasts. Checks skin for signs of irritation.		

	Abdomen: Folds bath blanket down so that it still covers pubic area. Washes abdomen, rinses, and pats dry. Covers with towel. Pulls bath blanket up to resident's chin. Removes towel.	
	Legs and Feet: Exposes one leg. Places a towel under it. Washes thigh. Uses long downward strokes. Rinses and pats dry. Does same from knee to ankle. Places another towel under foot. Moves basin to towel. Places foot into basin. Washes foot and between toes. Rinses foot and pats dry. Dries between toes. Gives nail care if assigned. Applies lotion to foot if ordered. Repeats steps for other leg and foot.	
	Back: Helps resident move to center of bed. Asks resident to turn onto his side. If bed has rails, raises rail on far side for safety. Folds blanket away from back. Places a towel lengthwise next to back. Washes back, neck, and buttocks with long, downward strokes. Rinses and pats dry. Applies lotion if ordered.	
12.	Places towel under buttocks and upper thighs. Helps resident turn onto his back. If resident is able to wash perineal area, places a basin of clean, warm water and a washcloth and towel within reach. Leaves room if resident desires. If resident has a urinary catheter in place, reminds him not to pull on it.	
13.	If resident cannot provide perineal care, puts on gloves first and provides privacy at all times.	

14.	Perineal area and buttocks: Changes bath water. Washes, rinses, and dries perineal area. Works from front to back (clean to dirty).	
	For a female resident: Washes perineum with soap and water from front to back. Uses single strokes. Does not wash from back to front. Uses a clean area of washcloth or clean washcloth for each stroke. First wipes center of perineum, then each side. Then spreads labia majora and wipes from front to back on each side. Rinses area in same way. Dries entire perineal area. Moves from front to back. Uses a blotting motion with towel. Asks resident to turn on her side. Washes, rinses, and dries buttocks and anal area. Cleans anal area without contaminating perineal area.	
	For a male resident: If resident is uncircumcised, pulls back foreskin first. Gently pushes skin towards base of penis. Holds penis by shaft. Washes in a circular motion from tip down to base. Uses a clean area of washcloth or clean washcloth for each stroke. Rinses penis. If resident is uncircumcised, gently returns foreskin to normal position. Washes scrotum and groin. Rinses and pats dry. Asks resident to turn on his side. Washes, rinses, and dries buttocks and anal area. Cleans anal area without contaminating perineal area.	
15.	Removes bath blanket. Removes and disposes of gloves properly.	
16.	Washes hands.	
17.	Provides deodorant.	

18.	Puts clean gown on resident. Assists with brushing or combing resident's hair.		
19.	Replaces bedding. Makes resident comfortable.		
20.	Returns bed to low position if raised. Ensures resident's safety. Returns side rails to ordered position. Removes privacy measures.		
21.	Empties, rinses, and wipes bath basin. Returns to proper storage.		
22.	Places soiled clothing and linens in proper containers.		
23.	Leaves call light within resident's reach.		
24.	Washes hands.		
25.	Is courteous and respectful at all times.		
26.	Reports any changes to nurse and documents procedure using facility guidelines.		

_____   _____
Date Reviewed   Instructor Signature

_____   _____
Date Performed   Instructor Signature

Shampooing a resident's hair in bed

		yes	no
1.	Identifies self by name. Identifies resident and greets resident by name.		
2.	Washes hands.		
3.	Explains procedure to resident. Speaks clearly, slowly, and directly. Maintains face-to-face contact whenever possible. Encourages resident to assist if possible.		
4.	Provides for resident's privacy with a curtain, screen, or door. Makes sure room is at a comfortable temperature and there are no drafts.		
5.	Practices good body mechanics. Adjusts bed to safe working level. Locks bed wheels.		
6.	Lowers head of bed. Removes pillow.		
7.	Tests water temperature with thermometer or wrist. Ensures it is safe. Has resident check water temperature. Adjusts if necessary.		
8.	Raises side rail farthest from self.		
9.	Places waterproof pad under resident's head and shoulders. Covers resident with bath blanket. Folds back top sheet and regular blankets.		
10.	Places collection container under resident's head. Places one towel across resident's shoulders.		
11.	Protects resident's eyes with dry washcloth.		
12.	Uses pitcher or attachment to wet hair thoroughly. Applies a small amount of shampoo, usually size of a quarter.		
13.	Lathers and massages scalp with fingertips. Uses a circular motion from front to back. Does not scratch scalp.		
14.	Rinses hair until water runs clear. Applies conditioner. Rinses as directed on container.		
15.	Covers resident's hair with clean towel. Dries his face with washcloth used to protect eyes.		
16.	Removes trough and waterproof covering.		
17.	Raises head of bed.		
18.	Gently rubs scalp and hair with towel.		
19.	Dries and combs resident's hair as he or she prefers.		
20.	Makes resident comfortable.		

21.	Returns bed to low position if raised. Ensures resident's safety. Returns side rails to ordered position. Removes privacy measures.		
22.	Empties, rinses, and wipes bath basin/pitcher. Returns to proper storage.		
23.	Cleans comb/brush. Returns hair dryer and comb/brush to proper storage.		
24.	Places soiled linen in proper container.		
25.	Leaves call light within resident's reach.		
26.	Washes hands.		
27.	Is courteous and respectful at all times.		
28.	Reports any changes to nurse and documents procedure using facility guidelines.		

_____   _____
Date Reviewed   Instructor Signature

_____   _____
Date Performed   Instructor Signature

Giving a shower or tub bath

		yes	no
1.	Washes hands.		
2.	Places equipment in shower or tub room. Cleans shower or tub area and shower chair.		
3.	Washes hands.		
4.	Goes to resident's room. Identifies self by name. Identifies resident and greets resident by name.		
5.	Explains procedure to resident. Speaks clearly, slowly, and directly. Maintains face-to-face contact whenever possible. Encourages resident to assist if possible.		

6.	Provides for resident's privacy with a curtain, screen, or door.		
7.	Helps resident to put on non-skid footwear. Transports resident to shower or tub room.		
	For a shower:		
8.	If using a shower chair, places it into position and locks its wheels. Safely transfers resident into shower chair.		
9.	Turns on water. Tests water temperature with thermometer. Has resident check water temperature.		
	For a tub bath:		
8.	Safely transfers resident onto chair or tub lift.		
9.	Fills tub halfway with warm water. Tests water temperature with thermometer. Has resident check water temperature.		
	Remaining steps for either procedure:		
10.	Puts on gloves.		
11.	Helps resident remove clothing and shoes.		
12.	Helps resident into shower or tub. Puts shower chair into shower and locks wheels.		
13.	Stays with resident during entire procedure.		
14.	Lets resident wash as much as possible on his or her own. Assists to wash his or her face.		
15.	Helps resident shampoo hair. Carefully sprays water over hair, taking care that water and shampoo/conditioner do not get into eyes. Rinses hair thoroughly.		
16.	Helps to wash and rinse entire body. Moves from head to toe (clean to dirty).		

Name: _____

17.	Turns off water or drains tub. Covers resident with bath blanket until tub drains.		
18.	Unlocks shower chair wheels if used. Rolls resident out of shower, or helps resident out of tub and onto a chair.		
19.	Gives resident towel(s) and helps to pat dry. Remembers to pat dry under breasts, between skin folds, in perineal area, and between toes.		
20.	Applies lotion and deodorant as needed.		
21.	Places soiled clothing and linens in proper containers.		
22.	Removes gloves and disposes of them properly.		
23.	Washes hands.		
24.	Helps resident dress and comb hair before leaving shower or tub room. Puts non-skid footwear on resident. Returns resident to room.		
25.	Makes resident comfortable.		
26.	Leaves call light within resident's reach.		
27.	Washes hands.		
28.	Is courteous and respectful at all times.		
29.	Reports any changes to nurse and documents procedure using facility guidelines.		

_____   _____
Date Reviewed   Instructor Signature

_____   _____
Date Performed   Instructor Signature

Giving a back rub

		yes	no
1.	Identifies self by name. Identifies resident and greets resident by name.		
2.	Washes hands.		

3.	Explains procedure to resident. Speaks clearly, slowly, and directly. Maintains face-to-face contact whenever possible. Encourages resident to assist if possible.		
4.	Provides for resident's privacy with a curtain, screen, or door.		
5.	Practices good body mechanics. Adjusts bed to safe working level. Locks bed wheels.		
6.	Lowers side rail on near side.		
7.	Positions resident lying on side or stomach. Covers with a bath blanket. Exposes back to top of buttocks.		
8.	Warms lotion by putting bottle in warm water for five minutes. Runs hands under warm water. Pours lotion on hands. Rubs them together.		
9.	Places hands on each side of upper part of buttocks. Makes long, smooth upward strokes with both hands. Moves along each side of spine, up to shoulders. Circles hands outward. Moves back along outer edges of back. At buttocks, makes another circle. Moves hands back up to shoulders. Repeats this motion for three to five minutes.		
10.	Kneads with first two fingers and thumb of each hand. Places them at base of spine. Moves upward together along each side of spine. Applies gentle downward pressure with fingers and thumbs. Follows same direction as with long smooth strokes, circling at shoulders and buttocks.		

Name: _____

11.	Gently massages bony areas. Uses circular motions of fingertips. If any of these areas are red, massages around them rather than on them.		
12.	Finishes with some long, smooth strokes.		
13.	Dries back if it has extra lotion remaining.		
14.	Removes bath blanket. Helps resident with getting dressed. Makes resident comfortable.		
15.	Returns bed to low position if raised. Ensures resident's safety. Returns side rails to ordered position. Removes privacy measures.		
16.	Stores supplies. Places soiled clothing and linens in proper containers.		
17.	Leaves call light within resident's reach.		
18.	Washes hands.		
19.	Is courteous and respectful at all times.		
20.	Reports any changes to nurse and documents procedure using facility guidelines.		

_____   _____
Date Reviewed   Instructor Signature

_____   _____
Date Performed   Instructor Signature

Providing oral care

		yes	no
1.	Identifies self by name. Identifies resident and greets resident by name.		
2.	Washes hands.		
3.	Explains procedure to resident. Speaks clearly, slowly, and directly. Maintains face-to-face contact whenever possible. Encourages resident to assist if possible.		
4.	Provides for resident's privacy with a curtain, screen, or door.		
5.	Practices good body mechanics. Adjusts bed to safe working level. Locks bed wheels. Makes sure resident is sitting upright.		
6.	Lowers side rail on near side.		
7.	Puts on gloves.		
8.	Places towel across resident's chest.		
9.	Wets brush. Puts on small amount of toothpaste.		
10.	Cleans entire mouth using gentle strokes. First brushes inner, outer and chewing surfaces of upper teeth, then does same with lower teeth. Uses short strokes. Brushes back and forth.		
11.	Holds emesis basin to resident's chin.		
12.	Has resident rinse mouth with water and spit into emesis basin.		
13.	Wipes resident's mouth and removes towel. Makes resident comfortable.		
14.	Returns bed to low position if raised. Ensures resident's safety. Returns side rails to ordered position. Removes privacy measures.		
15.	Empties, rinses and wipes emesis basin. Rinses toothbrush. Returns supplies to proper storage.		
16.	Disposes of soiled linen in proper container.		
17.	Removes and disposes of gloves properly.		
18.	Leaves call light within resident's reach.		
19.	Washes hands.		
20.	Is courteous and respectful at all times.		

Name: _____

21.	Reports any changes to nurse and documents procedure using facility guidelines.		

_____   _____
Date Reviewed   Instructor Signature

_____   _____
Date Performed   Instructor Signature

Flossing teeth

		yes	no
1.	Identifies self by name. Identifies resident and greets resident by name.		
2.	Washes hands.		
3.	Explains procedure to resident. Speaks clearly, slowly, and directly. Maintains face-to-face contact whenever possible. Encourages resident to assist if possible.		
4.	Provides for resident's privacy with a curtain, screen, or door.		
5.	Practices good body mechanics. Adjusts bed to safe working level. Locks bed wheels. Makes sure resident is in an upright sitting position.		
6.	Lowers side rail on near side.		
7.	Puts on gloves.		
8.	Wraps ends of floss securely around each index finger.		
9.	Starting with back teeth, places floss between teeth. Moves it down surface of tooth. Uses a gentle sawing motion. Continues to gum line. At gum line, curves floss into a letter C. Slips it gently into space between gum and tooth. Then goes back up, scraping that side of tooth. Repeats this on side of other tooth.		
10.	After every two teeth, unwinds floss from fingers. Uses a clean area. Flosses all teeth.		

11.	Offers water to rinse mouth. Asks resident to spit it into basin.		
12.	Offers resident a face towel when done flossing all teeth.		
13.	Returns bed to low position if raised. Ensures resident's safety. Returns side rails to ordered position. Removes privacy measures.		
14.	Cleans and returns supplies to proper storage.		
15.	Disposes of soiled linen in proper container.		
16.	Removes and disposes of gloves properly.		
17.	Leaves call light within resident's reach.		
18.	Washes hands.		
19.	Is courteous and respectful at all times.		
20.	Reports any changes to nurse and documents procedure using facility guidelines.		

_____   _____
Date Reviewed   Instructor Signature

_____   _____
Date Performed   Instructor Signature

Cleaning and storing dentures

		yes	no
1.	Identifies self by name. Identifies resident and greets resident by name.		
2.	Washes hands.		
3.	Explains procedure to resident. Speaks clearly, slowly, and directly. Maintains face-to-face contact whenever possible. Encourages resident to assist if possible.		
4.	Provides for resident's privacy with a curtain, screen, or door.		

5.	Practices good body mechanics. Adjusts bed to safe working level. Locks bed wheels. Makes sure resident is sitting upright.		
6.	Lowers side rail on near side.		
7.	Puts on gloves.		
8.	Lines sink/basin with towel(s) or fills sink 3/4 full with water. Handles dentures carefully.		
9.	Asks resident to sit upright.		
10.	Removes lower denture first. Grasps lower denture with a gauze square and removes it. Firmly grasps upper denture with a gauze square. Gives a slight downward pull to break suction. Turns it at an angle to take it out of mouth.		
11.	Rinses dentures in cool running water before brushing them. Does not use hot water.		
12.	Applies toothpaste or cleanser to toothbrush.		
13.	Brushes dentures on all surfaces.		
14.	Rinses all surfaces of dentures under cool running water.		
15.	Offers water to rinse resident's mouth. Asks resident to spit it into emesis basin.		
16.	Rinses denture cup if placing clean dentures inside it.		
17.	Places dentures in clean denture cup with solution or cool water and covers. Makes sure cup is labeled with resident's name. Returns denture cup to storage.		

18.	If replacing dentures in resident's mouth, makes sure resident is still sitting upright. Applies denture cream or adhesive to dentures if needed. When resident's mouth is open, places upper denture into mouth by turning it at an angle. Straightens it. Presses it onto upper gum line firmly and evenly. Inserts lower denture onto gum line of lower jaw. Presses firmly.		
19.	Returns bed to low position if raised. Ensures resident's safety. Returns side rails to ordered position. Removes privacy measures.		
20.	Cleans and returns equipment to proper storage.		
21.	Disposes of towels in appropriate container or drain sink.		
22.	Removes and disposes of gloves properly.		
23.	Leaves call light within resident's reach.		
24.	Washes hands.		
25.	Is courteous and respectful at all times.		
26.	Reports any changes in resident or appearance of dentures to nurse. Documents procedure using facility guidelines.		

_____ _____
Date Reviewed   Instructor Signature

_____ _____
Date Performed   Instructor Signature

Providing oral care for the unconscious resident

		yes	no
1.	Identifies self by name. Identifies resident and greets resident by name.		
2.	Washes hands.		

3.	Explains procedure to resident. Speaks clearly, slowly, and directly. Maintains face-to-face contact whenever possible.		
4.	Provides for resident's privacy with a curtain, screen, or door.		
5.	Practices good body mechanics. Adjusts bed to a safe level, usually waist high. Locks bed wheels.		
6.	Lowers side rail on near side.		
7.	Puts on gloves.		
8.	Turns resident's head to side. Places a towel under his cheek and chin. Places an emesis basin next to cheek and chin for excess fluid.		
9.	Holds mouth open with tongue depressor.		
10.	Dips swab in cleaning solution. Wipes inner, outer, and chewing surfaces of upper and lower teeth, gums, tongue, and inside surfaces of mouth. Changes swab often. Repeats until mouth is clean.		
11.	Rinses with clean swab dipped in water.		
12.	Removes towel and basin. Pats lips or face dry if needed. Applies lip lubricant.		
13.	Returns bed to low position if raised. Ensures resident's safety. Returns side rails to ordered position. Removes privacy measures.		
14.	Cleans and returns supplies to proper storage.		
15.	Disposes of soiled linen in proper container.		
16.	Removes and disposes of gloves properly.		
17.	Leaves call light within resident's reach.		
18.	Washes hands.		

| 19. | Is courteous and respectful at all times. | | |
| 20. | Reports any changes in resident to nurse. Reports any problems with teeth, mouth, tongue, and lips to nurse. Documents procedure using facility guidelines. | | |

_____ _____
Date Reviewed   Instructor Signature

_____ _____
Date Performed   Instructor Signature

Shaving a resident

		yes	no
1.	Identifies self by name. Identifies resident and greets resident by name.		
2.	Washes hands.		
3.	Explains procedure to resident. Speaks clearly, slowly, and directly. Maintains face-to-face contact whenever possible. Encourages resident to assist if possible.		
4.	Provides for resident's privacy with a curtain, screen, or door.		
5.	Practices good body mechanics. Adjusts bed to safe working level. Locks bed wheels.		
6.	Lowers side rail on near side.		
7.	Raises head of bed so resident is sitting up.		
	Shaving using a safety or disposable razor:		
8.	Fills bath basin halfway with warm water.		
9.	Drapes towel under resident's chin.		
10.	Applies gloves.		
11.	Moistens beard with warm washcloth. Puts shaving cream or soap over area.		

12.	Holds skin taut. Shaves beard in downward, short and even strokes on face and upward strokes on neck. Rinses razor often in warm water to keep it clean and wet.		
	Shaving using an electric razor:		
8	Does not use electric razor near water or if oxygen is in use or resident has pacemaker		
9	Drapes towel under resident's chin		
10	Applies gloves.		
11	Applies pre-shave lotion as resident wishes		
12	Holds skin taut. Shaves with smooth, even movements. Shaves beard with back and forth motion in direction of beard growth with foil shaver. Shaves beard in circular motion with three-head shaver.		
13.	Offers mirror to resident.		
14.	Washes, rinses, and dries face after shave. Applies after-shave lotion if requested.		
15.	Removes towel.		
16.	Removes and disposes of gloves properly. Washes hands.		
	Final steps:		
17.	Makes sure that resident and environment are free of loose hairs. Makes resident comfortable.		
18.	Returns bed to low position if raised. Ensures resident's safety. Returns side rails to ordered position. Removes privacy measures.		

19.	For safety razor: Rinses safety razor. For disposable razor: Disposes of a disposable razor in biohazard container. For electric razor: Cleans head of electric razor. Removes whiskers from razor. Recaps shaving head. Returns razor to case.		
20.	Returns supplies and equipment to proper storage.		
21.	Disposes of soiled linen in proper container.		
22.	Leaves call light within resident's reach.		
23.	Washes hands.		
24.	Is courteous and respectful at all times.		
25.	Reports any changes to nurse and documents procedure using facility guidelines.		

_____   _____
Date Reviewed   Instructor Signature

_____   _____
Date Performed   Instructor Signature

Providing fingernail care

		yes	no
1.	Identifies self by name. Identifies resident and greets resident by name.		
2.	Washes hands.		
3.	Explains procedure to resident. Speaks clearly, slowly, and directly. Maintains face-to-face contact whenever possible. Encourages resident to assist if possible.		
4.	Provides for resident's privacy with a curtain, screen, or door.		
5.	Practices good body mechanics. If resident is in bed, adjusts bed to safe working level. Locks bed wheels.		
6.	Lowers side rail on side nearest self.		

Name: _____

7.	Fills basin halfway with warm water. Tests water temperature with thermometer or wrist. Ensures it is safe. Has resident check water temperature. Adjusts if necessary.		
8.	Places basin at a comfortable level for resident. Soaks resident's nails in basin. Soaks all ten fingertips for at least five minutes.		
9.	Removes hands. Washes hands with soapy washcloth, then rinses. Pats hands dry with towel, including between fingers.		
10.	Puts on gloves.		
11.	Places resident's hands on towel. Gently uses pointed end of orangewood stick to remove dirt from under nails.		
12.	Wipes orangewood stick on towel after each nail. Washes resident's hands again. Dries them thoroughly.		
13.	Grooms nails with file or emery board. Files in a curve.		
14.	Finishes with nails smooth and free of rough edges.		
15.	Applies lotion from fingertips to wrists. Makes resident comfortable.		
16.	Returns bed to low position if raised. Ensures resident's safety. Returns side rails to ordered position. Removes privacy measures.		
17.	Empties, rinses, and wipes basin. Returns to proper storage.		
18.	Disposes of soiled linen in proper container.		
19.	Removes and disposes of gloves properly.		
20.	Leaves call light within resident's reach.		
21.	Washes hands.		

22.	Is courteous and respectful at all times.		
23.	Reports any changes to nurse and documents procedure using facility guidelines.		

_____	_____
Date Reviewed	Instructor Signature
_____	_____
Date Performed	Instructor Signature

Combing or brushing hair

		yes	no
1.	Identifies self by name. Identifies resident and greets resident by name.		
2.	Washes hands.		
3.	Explains procedure to resident. Speaks clearly, slowly, and directly. Maintains face-to-face contact whenever possible. Encourages resident to assist if possible.		
4.	Provides for resident's privacy with a curtain, screen, or door.		
5.	Practices good body mechanics. If resident is in bed, adjusts bed to safe working level. Locks bed wheels.		
6.	Lowers side rail on near side.		
7.	Raises head of bed so resident is sitting up. Places a towel under head or around shoulders.		
8.	Removes any hair pins, hair ties and clips.		
9.	Removes tangles first by dividing hair into small sections. Gently combs out from ends of hair to scalp.		
10.	After tangles are removed, brushes two-inch sections of hair at a time. Brushes from roots to ends.		
11.	Neatly styles hair as resident prefers. Avoids childish hairstyles. Offers mirror to resident.		

12.	Makes resident comfortable.		
13.	Returns bed to low position if raised. Ensures resident's safety. Returns side rails to ordered position. Removes privacy measures.		
14.	Returns supplies to proper storage. Cleans hair from brush/comb. Cleans comb and brush.		
15.	Disposes of soiled linen in proper container.		
16.	Leaves call light within resident's reach.		
17.	Washes hands.		
18.	Is courteous and respectful at all times.		
19.	Reports any changes to nurse and documents procedure using facility guidelines.		

_____   _____
Date Reviewed   Instructor Signature

_____   _____
Date Performed   Instructor Signature

Dressing a resident

		yes	no
1.	Identifies self by name. Identifies resident and greets resident by name.		
2.	Washes hands.		
3.	Explains procedure to resident. Speaks clearly, slowly, and directly. Maintains face-to-face contact whenever possible. Encourages resident to assist if possible.		
4.	Provides for resident's privacy with a curtain, screen, or door.		
5.	Asks resident what she would like to wear. Dresses her in outfit of choice.		
6.	Removes resident's gown. Does not completely expose resident. Takes off stronger, or unaffected, side first when undressing.		

7.	Gathers up sleeve to ease pulling over affected arm. Inserts hand through sleeve and grasps resident's hand to support arm while dressing. Assists resident to put affected/weak arm through right sleeve of shirt, sweater, or slip before placing garment on unaffected arm.		
8.	Helps resident to put on skirt, pants, or dress. Puts affected/weak leg through skirt or pants first. Raises buttocks or turns resident from side to side to draw pants over buttocks up to waist.		
9.	Places bed at a safe level for resident, usually lowest position.		
10.	Applies socks, pulling them up until they are both smooth and without wrinkles. Applies non-skid footwear. Ties laces.		
11.	Finishes with resident dressed appropriately. Makes sure clothing is right-side out and zippers/buttons are fastened.		
12.	Removes privacy measures.		
13.	Places gown in soiled linen container.		
14.	Leaves call light within resident's reach.		
15.	Washes hands.		
16.	Is courteous and respectful at all times.		
17.	Reports any changes to nurse and documents procedure using facility guidelines.		

_____   _____
Date Reviewed   Instructor Signature

_____   _____
Date Performed   Instructor Signature

186

Measuring and recording oral temperature		
	yes	no
1.	Identifies self by name. Identifies resident and greets resident by name.		
2.	Washes hands.		
3.	Explains procedure to resident. Speaks clearly, slowly, and directly. Maintains face-to-face contact whenever possible. Encourages resident to assist if possible.		
4.	Provides for resident's privacy with a curtain, screen, or door.		
5.	Puts on gloves.		
Using a mercury-free glass thermometer:		
6.	Holds thermometer by stem.		
7.	Before inserting thermometer in resident's mouth, shakes thermometer down to below lowest number.		
8.	Puts on disposable sheath, if applicable. Gently inserts bulb end of thermometer into resident's mouth. Places it under tongue and to one side.		
9.	Tells resident to hold thermometer in mouth with lips closed. Assists as necessary. Asks resident not to bite down or to talk.		
10.	Leaves thermometer in place for at least three minutes.		
11.	Removes thermometer. Wipes with tissue from stem to bulb or removes sheath. Disposes of tissue or sheath.		
12.	Holds thermometer at eye level. Reads temperature. Remembers temperature reading.		
13.	Cleans thermometer according to facility policy. Returns it to plastic case or container. Stores it away from any heat source.		
Using a digital thermometer:		

6.	Puts on disposable sheath.		
7.	Turns on thermometer. Waits until "ready" sign appears.		
8.	Inserts end of digital thermometer into resident's mouth. Places under tongue and to one side.		
9.	Leaves in place until thermometer blinks or beeps.		
10.	Removes thermometer.		
11.	Reads temperature on display screen. Remembers temperature reading.		
12.	Using a tissue, removes and disposes of sheath.		
13.	Cleans thermometer according to facility policy. Replaces thermometer in case.		
Using an electronic thermometer:		
6.	Removes probe from base unit.		
7.	Puts on probe cover.		
8.	Inserts covered probe into resident's mouth. Places under tongue and to one side.		
9.	Leaves in place until tone is heard or steady or flashing light is seen.		
10.	Reads temperature on display screen. Remembers temperature reading.		
11.	Removes probe.		
12.	Presses eject button to discard cover.		
13.	Returns probe to holder.		
Final steps for all methods:		
14.	Removes privacy measures. Makes resident comfortable.		
15.	Removes and disposes of gloves properly.		
16.	Leaves call light within resident's reach.		
17.	Washes hands.		
18.	Is courteous and respectful at all times.		

19.	Reports any changes to nurse and documents procedure using facility guidelines. Records resident's name, temperature, date, time, and method used (oral).		

Date Reviewed	Instructor Signature

Date Performed	Instructor Signature

Measuring and recording rectal temperature		yes	no
1.	Identifies self by name. Identifies resident and greets resident by name.		
2.	Washes hands.		
3.	Explains procedure to resident. Speaks clearly, slowly, and directly. Maintains face-to-face contact whenever possible. Encourages resident to assist if possible.		
4.	Provides for resident's privacy with a curtain, screen, or door.		
5.	Practices good body mechanics. Adjusts bed to safe working level, usually waist high. Locks bed wheels.		
6.	Lowers side rail on side nearest self.		
7.	Helps resident to left-lying (Sims') position.		
8.	Folds back linens to expose only rectal area.		
9.	Puts on gloves.		
10.	**Mercury-free glass thermometer**: Holds thermometer by stem. Shakes thermometer down to below lowest number. Puts on disposable sheath. Applies small amount of lubricant to sheath.		
	Digital thermometer: Puts on disposable sheath. Applies small amount of lubricant to sheath. Turns on thermometer. Waits until "ready" sign appears.		
	Electronic thermometer: Removes probe from base unit. Puts on probe cover. Applies small amount of lubricant to cover.		
11.	Separates buttocks. Gently inserts thermometer one inch into rectum. Stops if meets resistance.		
12.	Replaces sheet over buttocks. Holds onto thermometer at all times.		
13.	**Mercury-free glass thermometer**: Holds thermometer in place for at least three minutes.		
	Digital thermometer: Holds thermometer in place until thermometer blinks or beeps.		
	Electronic thermometer: Leaves in place until tone is heard or steady or flashing light is seen.		
14.	Gently removes thermometer. Wipes with tissue from stem to bulb or removes sheath or cover. Disposes of tissue.		
15.	Reads thermometer. Remembers temperature reading.		
16.	**Mercury-free glass thermometer**: Cleans thermometer according to facility policy. Returns it to plastic case or container.		
	Digital thermometer: Discards sheath. Cleans thermometer according to facility policy. Returns thermometer to storage area.		
	Electronic thermometer: Discards cover. Returns probe to holder.		
17.	Removes and disposes of gloves properly. Washes hands.		
18.	Makes resident comfortable.		

19.	Returns bed to low position if raised. Ensures resident's safety. Returns side rails to ordered position. Removes privacy measures.		
20.	Leaves call light within resident's reach.		
21.	Washes hands.		
22.	Is courteous and respectful at all times.		
23.	Reports any changes to nurse and documents procedure using facility guidelines. Records resident's name, temperature, date, time, and method used (rectal).		

_____   _____
Date Reviewed   Instructor Signature

_____   _____
Date Performed   Instructor Signature

Measuring and recording tympanic temperature

		yes	no
1.	Identifies self by name. Identifies resident and greets resident by name.		
2.	Washes hands.		
3.	Explains procedure to resident. Speaks clearly, slowly, and directly. Maintains face-to-face contact whenever possible. Encourages resident to assist if possible.		
4.	Provides for resident's privacy with a curtain, screen, or door.		
5.	Puts on gloves.		
6.	Puts a disposable sheath over earpiece of thermometer.		
7.	Positions resident's head so that ear is in front. Straightens ear canal by pulling up and back on outside edge of ear. Inserts covered probe into ear canal. Presses button.		

8.	Holds thermometer in place until thermometer blinks or beeps.		
9.	Reads temperature. Remembers temperature reading. (Repeats procedure if reading seems too low.)		
10.	Disposes of sheath. Returns thermometer to storage or to battery charger if thermometer is rechargeable.		
11.	Makes resident comfortable.		
12.	Removes privacy measures.		
13.	Removes and disposes of gloves properly.		
14.	Leaves call light within resident's reach.		
15.	Washes hands.		
16.	Is courteous and respectful at all times.		
17.	Reports any changes to nurse and documents procedure using facility guidelines. Records resident's name, temperature, date, time, and method used (tympanic).		

_____   _____
Date Reviewed   Instructor Signature

_____   _____
Date Performed   Instructor Signature

Measuring and recording axillary temperature

		yes	no
1.	Identifies self by name. Identifies resident and greets resident by name.		
2.	Washes hands.		
3.	Explains procedure to resident. Speaks clearly, slowly, and directly. Maintains face-to-face contact whenever possible. Encourages resident to assist if possible.		
4.	Provides for resident's privacy with a curtain, screen, or door.		

Name: _____

#			
5.	Practices good body mechanics. Adjusts bed to safe working level. Locks bed wheels.		
6.	Puts on gloves.		
7.	Removes resident's arm from sleeve of gown. Wipes axillary area with tissues.		
8.	**Mercury-free glass thermometer**: Holds thermometer by stem. Shakes thermometer down to below lowest number. Puts on disposable sheath, if applicable.		
	Digital thermometer: Puts on disposable sheath. Turns on thermometer. Waits until "ready" sign appears.		
	Electronic thermometer: Removes probe from base unit. Puts on probe cover.		
9.	Places end of thermometer in center of armpit. Folds resident's arm over chest.		
10.	**Mercury-free glass thermometer**: Holds thermometer in place, with arm close against side, for 10 minutes.		
	Digital thermometer: Holds thermometer in place until thermometer blinks or beeps.		
	Electronic thermometer: Leaves in place until tone is heard or steady or flashing light is seen.		
11.	Gently removes thermometer. Wipes with tissue from stem to bulb or removes sheath or cover. Disposes of tissue.		
12.	Reads thermometer. Remembers temperature reading.		
13.	**Mercury-free glass thermometer**: Cleans thermometer according to facility policy. Returns it to container for used thermometers.		

#			
	Digital thermometer: Discards sheath. Cleans thermometer according to facility policy. Returns thermometer to storage area.		
	Electronic thermometer: Discards cover. Returns probe to holder.		
14.	Puts resident's arm back into sleeve of gown. Makes resident comfortable.		
15.	Returns bed to low position. Ensures resident's safety. Returns side rails to ordered position. Removes privacy measures.		
16.	Removes and disposes of gloves properly.		
17.	Leaves call light within resident's reach.		
18.	Washes hands.		
19.	Is courteous and respectful at all times.		
20.	Reports any changes to nurse and documents procedure using facility guidelines. Records resident's name, temperature, date, time, and method used (axillary).		

_____   _____
Date Reviewed   Instructor Signature

_____   _____
Date Performed   Instructor Signature

Measuring and recording radial pulse and counting and recording respirations			
		yes	no
1.	Identifies self by name. Identifies resident and greets resident by name.		
2.	Washes hands.		

Name: _____

3.	Explains procedure to resident. Speaks clearly, slowly, and directly. Maintains face-to-face contact whenever possible. Encourages resident to assist if possible.		
4.	Provides for resident's privacy with a curtain, screen, or door.		
5.	Places fingertips on thumb side of resident's wrist to locate pulse.		
6.	Counts beats for one full minute.		
7.	Keeps fingertips on resident's wrist. Counts respirations for one full minute. Observes pattern and character of breathing.		
8.	Removes privacy measures. Makes resident comfortable.		
9.	Leaves call light within resident's reach.		
10.	Washes hands.		
11.	Is courteous and respectful at all times.		
12.	Reports any changes to nurse and documents procedure using facility guidelines. Records pulse rate, date, time and method used (radial). Records respiratory rate and pattern or character of breathing.		

Date Reviewed		Instructor Signature
Date Performed		Instructor Signature

Measuring and recording apical pulse		
		yes	no
1.	Identifies self by name. Identifies resident and greets resident by name.		
2.	Washes hands.		

3.	Explains procedure to resident. Speaks clearly, slowly, and directly. Maintains face-to-face contact whenever possible. Encourages resident to assist if possible.		
4.	Provides for resident's privacy with a curtain, screen, or door.		
5.	Practices good body mechanics. Adjusts bed to safe working level, usually waist high. Locks bed wheels.		
6.	Lowers side rail on near side.		
7.	Before using stethoscope, wipes diaphragm and earpieces with alcohol wipes.		
8.	Fits earpieces of stethoscope snugly in ears. Places flat metal diaphragm on left side of chest, just below nipple. Listens for heartbeat.		
9.	Uses second hand of watch to count beats for one full minute. Leaves stethoscope in place to count respirations.		
10.	Cleans earpieces and diaphragm of stethoscope with alcohol wipes. Stores stethoscope.		
11.	Makes resident comfortable.		
12.	Returns bed to low position. Ensures resident's safety. Returns side rails to ordered position. Removes privacy measures.		
13.	Leaves call light within resident's reach.		
14.	Washes hands.		
15.	Is courteous and respectful at all times.		

Name: _____

16.	Reports any changes to nurse and documents procedure using facility guidelines. Records pulse rate, date, time, and method used (apical). Notes any differences in rhythm.		

_____ _____
Date Reviewed   Instructor Signature

_____ _____
Date Performed   Instructor Signature

Measuring and recording apical-radial pulse

		yes	no
1.	Identifies self by name. Identifies resident and greets resident by name.		
2.	Washes hands.		
3.	Explains procedure to resident. Speaks clearly, slowly, and directly. Maintains face-to-face contact whenever possible. Encourages resident to assist if possible.		
4.	Provides for resident's privacy with a curtain, screen, or door.		
5.	Practices good body mechanics. Adjusts bed to safe working level. Locks bed wheels.		
6.	Lowers side rail on near side.		
7.	Before using stethoscope, wipes diaphragm and earpieces with alcohol wipes.		
8.	Fits earpieces of stethoscope snugly in ears. Places flat metal diaphragm on left side of chest, just below nipple. Listens for heartbeat.		
9.	Co-worker places fingertips on thumb side of resident's wrist to locate radial pulse.		

10.	After both pulses have been located, looks at second hand of watch. When second hand reaches "12" or "6," says, "Start," and both count beats for one full minute. Says, "Stop" after one minute.		
11.	Cleans earpieces and diaphragm of stethoscope with alcohol wipes. Stores stethoscope.		
12.	Makes resident comfortable.		
13.	Returns bed to low position. Ensures resident's safety. Returns side rails to ordered position. Removes privacy measures.		
14.	Leaves call light within resident's reach.		
15.	Washes hands.		
16.	Is courteous and respectful at all times.		
17.	Reports any changes to nurse and documents procedure using facility guidelines. Records both pulse rates, date, time, and method used (apical-radial). Records pulse deficit, if any. Notes any differences in rhythm.		

_____ _____
Date Reviewed   Instructor Signature

_____ _____
Date Performed   Instructor Signature

Measuring and recording blood pressure (one-step method)

		yes	no
1.	Identifies self by name. Identifies resident and greets resident by name.		
2.	Washes hands.		
3.	Explains procedure to resident. Speaks clearly, slowly, and directly. Maintains face-to-face contact whenever possible. Encourages resident to assist if possible.		

Name: _____

4.	Provides for resident's privacy with a curtain, screen, or door.		
5.	Positions resident's arm with palm up, level with the heart. Rolls up long sleeves approximately five inches above elbow.		
6.	With valve open, squeezes cuff. Makes sure it is completely deflated.		
7.	Places blood pressure cuff snugly on resident's upper arm.		
8.	Before using stethoscope, wipes diaphragm and earpieces with alcohol wipes.		
9.	Locates brachial pulse with fingertips.		
10.	Places diaphragm of stethoscope over brachial artery.		
11.	Places earpieces of stethoscope in ears.		
12.	Closes valve (clockwise) until it stops. Does not over-tighten it.		
13.	Inflates cuff to 30 mm Hg above point at which pulse is last heard.		
14.	Opens valve slightly with thumb and index finger. Deflates cuff slowly.		
15.	Watches gauge. Listens for sound of pulse.		
16.	Remembers reading at which first clear pulse sound is heard.		
17.	Continues listening for a change or muffling of pulse sound. Remembers this reading.		
18.	Opens valve. Deflates cuff completely. Removes cuff.		
19.	Wipes diaphragm and earpieces of stethoscope with alcohol. Stores equipment.		
20.	Makes resident comfortable. Removes privacy measures.		
21.	Leaves call light within resident's reach.		
22.	Washes hands.		

23.	Is courteous and respectful at all times.		
24.	Reports any changes to nurse and documents procedure using facility guidelines. Records both systolic and diastolic pressures.		

_____   _____
Date Reviewed   Instructor Signature

_____   _____
Date Performed   Instructor Signature

Measuring and recording blood pressure (two-step method)

		yes	no
1.	Identifies self by name. Identifies resident and greets resident by name.		
2.	Washes hands.		
3.	Explains procedure to resident. Speaks clearly, slowly, and directly. Maintains face-to-face contact whenever possible. Encourages resident to assist if possible.		
4.	Provides for resident's privacy with a curtain, screen, or door.		
5.	Positions resident's arm with palm up, level with the heart. Rolls up long sleeves approximately five inches above elbow.		
6.	With valve open, squeezes cuff. Makes sure it is completely deflated.		
7.	Places blood pressure cuff snugly on resident's upper arm. Places center of cuff over brachial artery.		
8.	Locates radial (wrist) pulse with fingertips.		
9.	Closes valve (clockwise) until it stops. Inflates cuff slowly, watching gauge.		
10.	Stops inflating when can no longer feel pulse. Notes reading.		
11.	Opens valve. Deflates cuff completely.		

12.	Writes down estimated systolic reading.		
13.	Before using stethoscope, wipes diaphragm and earpieces of stethoscope with alcohol wipes.		
14.	Locates brachial pulse with fingertips.		
15.	Places diaphragm of stethoscope over brachial artery.		
16.	Places earpieces of stethoscope in ears.		
17.	Closes valve (clockwise) until it stops. Does not over-tighten it.		
18.	Inflates cuff to 30 mm Hg above estimated systolic pressure.		
19.	Opens valve slightly with thumb and index finger. Deflates cuff slowly.		
20.	Watches gauge. Listens for sound of pulse.		
21.	Remembers reading at which first clear pulse sound is heard.		
22.	Continues listening for a change or muffling of pulse sound. Remembers reading.		
23.	Opens valve. Deflates cuff completely. Removes cuff.		
24.	Wipes diaphragm and earpieces of stethoscope with alcohol. Stores equipment.		
25.	Makes resident comfortable. Removes privacy measures.		
26.	Leaves call light within resident's reach.		
27.	Washes hands.		
28.	Is courteous and respectful at all times.		
29	Reports any changes to nurse and documents procedure using facility guidelines. Records both systolic and diastolic pressures.		

_____   _____
Date Reviewed   Instructor Signature

_____   _____
Date Performed   Instructor Signature

Feeding a resident who cannot feed self

		yes	no
1.	Identifies self by name. Identifies resident and greets resident by name.		
2.	Washes hands.		
3.	Explains procedure to resident. Speaks clearly, slowly, and directly. Maintains face-to-face contact whenever possible. Encourages resident to assist if possible.		
4.	Provides for resident's privacy with a curtain, screen, or door.		
5.	Picks up diet card. Verifies that resident has received correct tray.		
6.	Helps resident to wash hands (and face if needed) if resident cannot do it on her own.		
7.	Adjusts bed height to sit at resident's eye level. Locks bed wheels.		
8.	Lowers side rail on near side.		
9.	Raises head of bed. Makes sure resident is in an upright sitting position (at a 90-degree angle).		
10.	Helps resident to put on clothing protector, if desired.		
11.	Sits facing resident. Sits at resident's eye level. Sits on stronger side if resident has one-sided weakness.		
12.	Offers drink of beverage. Offers different types of food, allowing for resident's preferences. Does not feed all of one type before offering another type.		
13.	Offers food in bite-sized pieces. Reports any swallowing problems to nurse immediately. If resident has one-sided weakness, directs food to unaffected, or stronger, side.		
14.	Makes sure resident's mouth is empty before next bite or sip.		

Name: _____

		yes	no
15.	Offers beverage to resident throughout meal.		
16.	Talks with resident during meal.		
17.	Uses washcloths to wipe food from resident's mouth and hands as needed during meal. Wipes again at end of meal.		
18.	Removes clothing protector if used. Disposes of protector in proper container.		
19.	Removes food tray. Checks for eyeglasses, dentures, hearing aids, or any personal items before removing tray.		
20.	Makes resident comfortable.		
21.	Returns bed to low position. Ensures resident's safety. Returns side rails to ordered position. Removes privacy measures.		
22.	Leaves call light within resident's reach.		
23.	Washes hands.		
24.	Is courteous and respectful at all times.		
25.	Reports any changes to nurse and documents procedure using facility guidelines. Records intake of solid food and fluids properly.		

_____   _____
Date Reviewed   Instructor Signature

_____   _____
Date Performed   Instructor Signature

Measuring and recording intake and output

	Measuring intake:	yes	no
1.	Identifies self by name. Identifies resident and greets resident by name.		
2.	Washes hands.		

		yes	no
3.	Explains procedure to resident. Speaks clearly, slowly, and directly. Maintains face-to-face contact whenever possible. Encourages resident to assist if possible.		
4.	Provides for resident's privacy with a curtain, screen, or door.		
5.	Uses a graduate to measure fluid served and records measurement.		
6.	When resident has finished, measures any leftover fluids and notes amount.		
7.	Subtracts leftover amount from amount served and converts to mL.		
8.	Records time and amount of fluid consumed (in mL) in input column on I&O sheet.		
9.	Washes hands.		
	Measuring output:		
1.	Washes hands.		
2.	Puts on gloves before handling bedpan/urinal.		
3.	Pours contents of bedpan or urinal into measuring container without spilling or splashing.		
4.	Places container on flat surface and measures amount of urine at eye level, keeping container level.		
5.	Empties measuring container into toilet without splashing.		
6.	Rinses measuring container and pours rinse water into toilet. Cleans container using facility guidelines.		
7.	Rinses bedpan/urinal and pours rinse water into toilet. Uses approved disinfectant.		
8.	Returns bedpan/urinal and measuring container to proper storage.		
9.	Removes and disposes of gloves.		

10.	Washes hands before recording output.		
11.	Records contents of container in output column on sheet. Reports any changes to nurse.		

_____   _____
Date Reviewed   Instructor Signature

_____   _____
Date Performed   Instructor Signature

Assisting a resident with use of a bedpan			
		yes	no
1.	Identifies self by name. Identifies resident and greets resident by name.		
2.	Washes hands.		
3.	Explains procedure to resident. Speaks clearly, slowly, and directly. Maintains face-to-face contact whenever possible. Encourages resident to assist if possible.		
4.	Provides for resident's privacy with a curtain, screen, or door.		
5.	Before placing bedpan, lowers head of bed. Locks bed wheels.		
6.	Lowers side rail on near side. Makes sure far side rail is raised.		
7.	Applies gloves.		
8.	Covers resident with bath blanket, asks him to hold it, and pulls down top covers underneath. Does not expose more of resident than is needed.		

9.	Places disposable bed protector under resident's buttocks and hips. If resident cannot turn self, turns resident away from self. Ensures that resident cannot roll off bed. Places bed protector on area where resident will lie on back. Side of protector nearest resident is fanfolded and tucked under resident. Asks resident to roll onto back, or assists him to roll onto back if he is unable. Unfolds rest of bed protector so it completely covers area under and around resident's hips.		
10.	Asks resident to remove undergarments or help him to do so.		
11.	Asks resident to raise hips by pushing with feet and hands. Places bedpan correctly under resident's buttocks, avoiding trauma or pain.		
	Standard bedpan: Positions bedpan so wider end of pan is aligned with resident's buttocks. Fracture pan: Positions bedpan with handle toward foot of bed.		
	If resident cannot help in any way, keeps bed flat and rolls resident away from self. Slips bedpan under hips and rolls him back onto bedpan.		
12.	Raises head of bed after placing bedpan under resident. Raises side rail if bed has one.		
13.	Puts toilet tissue within resident's reach.		
14.	Leaves call light within resident's reach while resident is using bedpan. Asks resident to signal when finished.		
15.	Remains outside curtain until called by resident. When called, returns and lowers head of bed.		
16.	Removes bedpan carefully without causing trauma or pain. Covers bedpan.		

Name: _____

17.	Provides perineal care if assistance is needed. Remembers to wipe from front to back.		
18.	Notes color, odor, amount and consistency of contents. Empties contents of bedpan into toilet.		
19.	Rinses bedpan and pours rinse water into toilet. Uses approved disinfectant if facility policy.		
20.	Removes and disposes of gloves properly.		
21.	Washes hands.		
22.	Puts on clean gloves.		
23.	Returns bedpan to proper storage.		
24.	Assists resident to wash hands after using bedpan. Disposes of soiled washcloth or wipes in proper container. Helps resident put on undergarment.		
25.	Removes and disposes of gloves properly. Washes hands.		
26.	Makes resident comfortable.		
27.	Returns bed to low position. Ensures resident's safety. Returns side rails to ordered position. Removes privacy measures.		
28.	Leaves call light within resident's reach.		
29.	Washes hands.		
30.	Is courteous and respectful at all times.		
31.	Reports any changes to nurse and documents procedure using facility guidelines.		

_____   _____
Date Reviewed   Instructor Signature

_____   _____
Date Performed   Instructor Signature

Assisting a male resident with a urinal

		yes	no
1.	Identifies self by name. Identifies resident and greets resident by name.		
2.	Washes hands.		
3.	Explains procedure to resident. Speaks clearly, slowly, and directly. Maintains face-to-face contact whenever possible. Encourages resident to assist if possible.		
4.	Provides for resident's privacy with a curtain, screen, or door.		
5.	Locks bed wheels. Applies gloves.		
6.	Places a protective pad under resident's buttocks and hips.		
7.	Hands urinal to resident or places urinal between resident's legs and positions penis inside urinal. Replaces bed covers.		
8.	Leaves call light within resident's reach while resident is using urinal. Asks resident to signal when finished.		
9.	Remains outside curtain until called by resident. When called, returns and removes urinal carefully.		
10.	Notes color, odor, amount, and qualities of contents. Empties contents into toilet.		
11.	Rinses urinal and pours rinse water into toilet. Uses approved disinfectant if facility policy. Returns to proper storage.		
12.	Removes and disposes of gloves properly. Washes hands.		
13.	Assists resident to wash hands. Disposes of soiled washcloth or wipes properly.		
14.	Makes resident comfortable.		
15.	Ensures resident's safety. Removes privacy measures.		

16.	Leaves call light within resident's reach.		
17.	Washes hands.		
18.	Is courteous and respectful at all times.		
19.	Reports any changes to nurse and documents procedure using facility guidelines.		

_____   _____
Date Reviewed   Instructor Signature

_____   _____
Date Performed   Instructor Signature

Helping a resident use a portable commode

		yes	no
1.	Identifies self by name. Identifies resident and greets resident by name.		
2.	Washes hands.		
3.	Explains procedure to resident. Speaks clearly, slowly, and directly. Maintains face-to-face contact whenever possible. Encourages resident to assist if possible.		
4.	Provides for resident's privacy with a curtain, screen, or door.		
5.	Practices good body mechanics. Adjusts bed to low position. Locks bed wheels. Locks commode wheels.		
6.	Helps resident out of bed and to portable commode. Makes sure resident is wearing non-skid shoes.		
7.	If needed, helps resident remove clothing and sit comfortably on toilet seat. Puts toilet tissue within reach.		
8.	Places bath blanket over resident's legs. Leaves call light within resident's reach. Asks resident to signal when finished.		
9.	When called, returns and applies gloves.		

10.	Gives perineal care if help is needed. Wipes from front to back.		
11.	Removes and disposes of gloves properly. Washes hands.		
12.	Assists resident to wash hands after using commode. Disposes of soiled washcloth or wipes properly.		
13.	Assists back to bed. Returns bed to proper position. Ensures resident's safety. Removes privacy measures.		
14.	Removes waste basin. Notes color, odor, amount and consistency of contents. Empties into toilet.		
15.	Rinses container and pours rinse water into toilet. Uses approved disinfectant if facility policy. Returns to proper storage.		
16.	Removes and disposes of gloves properly.		
17.	Leaves call light within resident's reach.		
18.	Washes hands.		
19.	Is courteous and respectful at all times.		
20.	Reports any changes to nurse and documents procedure using facility guidelines.		

_____   _____
Date Reviewed   Instructor Signature

_____   _____
Date Performed   Instructor Signature

Giving a cleansing enema

		yes	no
1.	Identifies self by name. Identifies resident and greets resident by name.		
2.	Washes hands.		

Name: _____

3.	Explains procedure to resident. Speaks clearly, slowly, and directly. Maintains face-to-face contact whenever possible. Encourages resident to assist if possible.		
4.	Provides for resident's privacy with a curtain, screen, or door.		
5.	Practices good body mechanics. Adjusts bed to safe working level. Locks bed wheels.		
6.	Raises side rail on far side of bed. Lowers near side rail.		
7.	Helps resident into Sims' position. Covers with a bath blanket.		
8.	Places IV pole beside bed. Raises side rail.		
9.	Clamps enema tube. Prepares enema solution. Adds specific additive, if ordered. Fills bag with 500-1000 mL of warm water (105°F) and swishes fluid to mix well.		
10.	Unclamps tube. Lets small amount of solution run through tubing to release air. Re-clamps tube.		
11.	Hangs bag on IV pole. Makes sure bottom of enema bag is not more than 12 inches above resident's anus.		
12.	Applies gloves.		
13.	Lowers side rail. Uncovers resident enough to expose anus only.		
14.	Places disposable bed protector under resident. Places bedpan close to resident's body.		
15.	Lubricates two to four inches of tip of tubing with lubricating jelly.		
16.	Asks resident to breathe deeply to relieve cramps during procedure.		

17.	Places one hand on upper buttock. Lifts to expose anus. Asks resident to take a deep breath and exhale. Using other hand, gently inserts tip of tubing two to four inches into rectum. Stops immediately if resistance is felt or if resident complains of pain. If this happens, clamps tube and tells nurse immediately.		
18.	Unclamps tubing. Allows solution to flow slowly into rectum. Asks resident to take slow, deep breaths. If resident complains of cramping, clamps tubing and stops for a couple of minutes. Encourages him or her to take as much of solution as possible.		
19.	Clamps tubing before bag is empty, when solution is almost gone. Gently removes tip from rectum. Places tip into enema bag. Does not contaminate self, resident, or bed linens.		
20.	Asks resident to hold solution inside as long as possible.		
21.	Helps resident to use bedpan, commode, or get to bathroom. If resident uses a commode or bathroom, applies robe and non-skid footwear. Lowers bed to an appropriate level for resident before resident gets up.		
22.	Places call light and toilet paper within resident's reach. If resident is using bathroom, asks him not to flush toilet when finished.		
23.	Leaves resident if possible. Asks him to signal when he's finished.		
24.	Discards disposable equipment. Cleans area.		
25.	Removes and disposes of gloves properly. Washes hands.		

26.	When resident is done, puts on clean gloves. Using washcloths, helps with perineal care as needed.		
27.	Removes bedpan. Covers bedpan. Removes disposable bed protector.		
28.	Calls nurse to observe enema results.		
29.	Empties and rinses bedpan. Pours rinse water into toilet. Uses approved disinfectant if facility policy. Returns to proper storage. Disposes of soiled washcloths.		
30.	Removes and disposes of gloves properly. Washes hands.		
31.	Helps resident wash hands.		
32.	Removes bath blanket. Makes resident comfortable.		
33.	Returns bed to low position if raised. Ensures resident's safety. Returns side rails to ordered position. Removes privacy measures.		
34.	Leaves call light within resident's reach.		
35.	Washes hands.		
36.	Is courteous and respectful at all times.		
37.	Reports any changes to nurse and documents procedure using facility guidelines.		

_____   _____
Date Reviewed   Instructor Signature

_____   _____
Date Performed   Instructor Signature

Giving a commercial enema

		yes	no
1.	Identifies self by name. Identifies resident and greets resident by name.		
2.	Washes hands.		

3.	Explains procedure to resident. Speaks clearly, slowly, and directly. Maintains face-to-face contact whenever possible. Encourages resident to assist if possible.		
4.	Provides for resident's privacy with a curtain, screen, or door.		
5.	Practices good body mechanics. Adjusts bed to safe working level. Locks bed wheels.		
6.	Raises side rail on far side of bed. Lowers near side rail.		
7.	Helps resident into left-sided Sims' position. Covers with a bath blanket.		
8.	Applies gloves.		
9.	Places disposable bed protector under resident. Places bedpan close to resident's body.		
10.	Uncovers resident enough to expose anus only.		
11.	Adds extra lubricating jelly to tip of bottle if needed.		
12.	Asks resident to breathe deeply to relieve cramps during procedure.		
13.	Places one hand on upper buttock. Lifts to expose anus. Asks resident to take a deep breath and exhale. Using other hand, gently inserts tip of tubing about one and a half inches into rectum. Stops immediately if resistance is felt or if resident complains of pain.		
14.	Slowly squeezes and rolls enema container so that solution runs inside resident. Stops when container is almost empty.		
15.	Gently removes tip from rectum, continuing to keep pressure on container until bottle is placed inside box upside down.		
16.	Asks resident to hold solution inside as long as possible.		

Name: _____

17.	Helps resident to use bedpan or commode, or get to bathroom. If resident uses a commode or bathroom, applies robe and non-skid footwear. Lowers bed to its lowest position before resident gets up.		
18.	Places call light and toilet paper within resident's reach. If resident is using bathroom, asks him not to flush toilet when finished.		
19.	Leaves resident if possible. Asks him to signal when he's finished.		
20.	Discards disposable equipment. Cleans area.		
21.	Removes and disposes of gloves properly. Washes hands.		
22.	When resident is done, puts on clean gloves. Using washcloths, helps with perineal care as needed.		
23.	Removes bedpan. Covers bedpan. Removes disposable bed protector. Calls nurse to observe enema results.		
24.	Empties bedpan. Rinses bedpan. Pours rinse water into toilet. Uses approved disinfectant if facility policy. Returns it to proper storage. Disposes of soiled washcloths properly.		
25.	Removes and disposes of gloves properly. Washes hands.		
26.	Helps resident wash hands.		
27.	Removes bath blanket. Makes resident comfortable.		
28.	Returns bed to low position. Ensures resident's safety. Returns side rails to ordered position. Removes privacy measures.		
29.	Leaves call light within resident's reach.		

30.	Washes hands.		
31.	Is courteous and respectful at all times.		
32.	Reports any changes to nurse and documents procedure using facility guidelines.		

_____   _____
Date Reviewed   Instructor Signature

_____   _____
Date Performed   Instructor Signature

Collecting a stool specimen

		yes	no
1.	Identifies self by name. Identifies resident and greets resident by name.		
2.	Washes hands.		
3.	Explains procedure to resident. Speaks clearly, slowly and directly. Maintains face-to-face contact whenever possible. Encourages resident to assist if possible.		
4.	Provides for resident's privacy with a curtain, screen or door..		
5.	Practices good body mechanics. Adjusts bed to safe working level. Locks bed wheels.		
6.	Lowers side rail on near side.		
7.	Puts on gloves.		
8.	Asks resident not to urinate at the same time as moving bowels and not to put toilet paper in with the sample. Provides plastic bag to discard toilet paper separately.		
9.	Fits specimen pan to toilet or provides resident with bedpan. Leaves the room and asks to resident to call when he is finished.		
10.	Helps as necessary with perineal care. Helps resident wash hands, and makes resident comfortable. Removes gloves.		

		yes	no
11.	Washes hands again.		
12.	Puts on clean gloves.		
13.	Uses tongue blades to take about two tablespoons of stool and puts it in container without touching the inside. Covers container tightly.		
14.	Disposes of tongue blades properly. Empties bedpan or container into toilet. Cleans and stores equipment properly.		
15.	Labels container.		
16.	Removes and disposes of gloves.		
17.	Makes resident comfortable.		
18.	Returns bed to proper position. Removes privacy measures.		
19.	Places call light within resident's reach.		
20.	Washes hands.		
21.	Reports changes in resident.		
22.	Documents procedure. Notes amount and characteristics of stool.		

_____ _____
Date Reviewed   Instructor Signature

_____ _____
Date Performed   Instructor Signature

		yes	no
6.	Flips tongue blade (or uses new tongue blade). Gets some stool from another part of specimen. Smears small amount of stool onto Box B of test card.		
7.	Closes test card. Turns over to other side.		
8.	Opens flap.		
9.	Opens developer. Applies developer to each box. Follows manufacturer's instructions.		
10.	Waits amount of time listed in instructions, usually between 10 and 60 seconds.		
11.	Watches squares for any color changes. Records color changes. Follows instructions.		
12.	Places tongue blade(s) and test packet in disposable bag.		
13.	Disposes of plastic bag properly in biohazard container.		
14.	Removes and disposes of gloves properly. Washes hands.		
15.	Reports any changes to nurse and documents procedure using facility guidelines.		

_____ _____
Date Reviewed   Instructor Signature

_____ _____
Date Performed   Instructor Signature

Testing a stool specimen for occult blood

		yes	no
1.	Washes hands.		
2.	Puts on gloves.		
3.	Opens test card.		
4.	Picks up a tongue blade. Gets small amount of stool from specimen container.		
5.	Using a tongue blade, smears a small amount of stool onto Box A of test card.		

Caring for an ostomy

		yes	no
1.	Identifies self by name. Identifies resident. Greets resident by name.		
2.	Washes hands.		
3.	Explains procedure to resident. Speaks clearly, slowly, and directly. Maintains face-to-face contact whenever possible. Encourages resident to assist if possible.		
4.	Provides for resident's privacy with a curtain, screen, or door.		

Name: _____

5.	Practices good body mechanics. Adjusts bed to safe working level. Locks bed wheels.		
6.	Lowers side rail on near side.		
7.	Places disposable bed protector under resident. Covers resident with bath blanket. Pulls down top sheet and blankets. Exposes only ostomy site. Offers resident a towel to keep clothing dry.		
8.	Puts on gloves.		
9.	Undoes ostomy belt if used. Pulls gently on one edge of ostomy appliance to release air.		
10.	Removes ostomy bag carefully. Places it in plastic bag. Notes color, odor, consistency, and amount of stool in bag.		
11.	Wipes area around stoma with gauze squares. Discards squares in plastic bag.		
12.	Adds small amount of mild soap or cleanser to warm water. Using a washcloth, washes area in one direction, away from stoma. Rinses. Pats dry with another towel. Applies skin barrier as ordered. Temporarily covers stoma opening with gauze squares.		
13.	Applies deodorant to bag if used. Removes gauze squares, and places in plastic bag. Puts clean ostomy appliance on resident. Holds in place and seals securely. Makes sure bottom of bag is clamped. Attaches to ostomy belt if used.		
14.	Removes and discards disposable bed protector. Places soiled linens in proper container.		
15.	Removes bag and gauze squares. Discards bag and squares in proper container.		
16.	Removes and disposes of gloves properly. Washes hands.		

17.	Makes resident comfortable.		
18.	Returns bed to low position. Ensures resident's safety. Returns side rails to ordered position. Removes privacy measures.		
19.	Leaves call light within resident's reach.		
20.	Washes hands.		
21.	Is courteous and respectful at all times.		
22.	Reports any changes to nurse and documents procedure using facility guidelines.		

_____   _____
Date Reviewed   Instructor Signature

_____   _____
Date Performed   Instructor Signature

Providing perineal care for an incontinent resident			
		yes	no
1.	Identifies self by name. Identifies resident and greets resident by name.		
2.	Washes hands.		
3.	Explains procedure to resident. Speaks clearly, slowly, and directly. Maintains face-to-face contact whenever possible. Encourages resident to assist if possible.		
4.	Provides for resident's privacy with a curtain, screen, or door.		
5.	Practices good body mechanics. Adjusts bed to safe working level. Locks bed wheels.		
6.	Lowers side rail on near side.		
7.	Lowers head of bed. Positions resident lying flat on his or her back.		

8.	Tests water temperature with thermometer or wrist. Ensures it is safe. Has resident check water temperature. Adjusts if necessary.		
9.	Puts on gloves.		
10.	Covers resident with bath blanket. Moves top linens to foot of bed.		
11.	Removes soiled bed protector from underneath resident by turning resident on his side, away from self. Rolls soiled pad into itself with wet side in/dry side out.		
12.	Places clean bed protector under resident's buttocks.		
13.	Returns resident to lying on his back.		
14.	Exposes perineal area only. Cleans perineal area.		
	For a female resident: Washes perineum with soap and water from front to back. Uses single strokes. Uses a clean area of washcloth or clean washcloth for each stroke. First wipes center of perineum, then each side. Spreads labia majora and wipes from front to back on each side. Rinses area in same way. Dries entire perineal area. Moves from front to back, using a blotting motion with towel. Asks resident to turn on side. Washes, rinses, and dries buttocks and anal area. Cleanses anal area without contaminating perineal area.		

	For a male resident: If resident is uncircumcised, retracts foreskin. Gently pushes skin towards base of penis. Holds penis by shaft and washes in a circular motion from tip down to base. Uses a clean area of washcloth or clean washcloth for each stroke. Rinses penis. If resident is uncircumcised, gently returns foreskin to normal position. Washes scrotum and groin. Rinses and pats dry. Asks resident to turn on side. Washes, rinses, and dries buttocks and anal area. Cleanses anal area without contaminating perineal area.		
15.	Turns resident on side away from self. Removes wet bed protector after drying buttocks.		
16.	Places a dry bed protector under resident.		
17.	Repositions resident.		
18.	Removes bath blanket. Replaces top covers. Makes resident comfortable.		
19.	Returns bed to low position. Ensures resident's safety. Returns side rails to ordered position. Removes privacy measures.		
20.	Empties, rinses, and wipes basin. Returns to proper storage.		
21.	Places soiled linens, clothing and bed protectors in proper containers.		
22.	Removes and disposes of gloves properly.		
23.	Leaves call light within resident's reach.		
24.	Washes hands.		
25.	Is courteous and respectful at all times.		

26.	Reports any changes to nurse and documents procedure using facility guidelines.		

Date Reviewed	Instructor Signature
Date Performed	Instructor Signature

Providing catheter care

		yes	no
1.	Identifies self by name. Identifies resident. Greets resident by name.		
2.	Washes hands.		
3.	Explains procedure to resident. Speaks clearly, slowly, and directly. Maintains face-to-face contact whenever possible. Encourages resident to assist if possible.		
4.	Provides for resident's privacy with a curtain, screen, or door.		
5.	Practices good body mechanics. Adjusts bed to safe working level. Locks bed wheels.		
6.	Lowers side rail on near side.		
7.	Lowers head of bed. Positions resident lying flat on back.		
8.	Removes or folds back top bedding. Keeps resident covered with bath blanket.		
9.	Tests water temperature with thermometer or wrist and ensures it is safe. Has resident check water temperature. Adjusts if necessary.		
10.	Puts on gloves.		
11.	Avoids contact with clothing and soiled pads or soiled linens throughout procedure.		
12.	Asks resident to flex her knees and raise buttocks off bed by pushing against mattress with feet. Places clean bed protector under buttocks.		

13.	Exposes only area necessary to clean catheter.		
14.	Places towel or pad under catheter tubing before washing.		
15.	Applies soap to wet washcloth. Cleans area around meatus. Uses a clean area of washcloth for each stroke.		
16.	Holds catheter near meatus. Avoids tugging catheter.		
17.	Cleans at least four inches of catheter nearest meatus. Moves in only one direction, away from meatus. Uses a clean area of cloth for each stroke.		
18.	Rinses area around meatus, using a clean area of washcloth for each stroke. Pats dry with clean cloth.		
19.	Rinses at least four inches of catheter nearest meatus. Moves in only one direction, away from meatus. Uses a clean area of cloth for each stroke.		
20.	Removes towel or pad from under catheter tubing.		
21.	Replaces top covers. Removes bath blanket. Makes resident comfortable.		
22.	Returns bed to low position. Ensures resident's safety. Returns side rails to ordered position. Removes privacy measures.		
23.	Empties, rinses, and wipes basin. Returns to proper storage.		
24.	Disposes of soiled linen in proper containers.		
25.	Removes and disposes of gloves properly.		
26.	Leaves call light within resident's reach.		
27	Washes hands.		

28.	Is courteous and respectful at all times.		
29.	Reports any changes to nurse and documents procedure using facility guidelines.		

_____   _____
Date Reviewed   Instructor Signature

_____   _____
Date Performed   Instructor Signature

Emptying a catheter drainage bag

		yes	no
1.	Identifies self by name. Identifies resident and greets resident by name.		
2.	Washes hands.		
3.	Explains procedure to resident. Speaks clearly, slowly, and directly. Maintains face-to-face contact whenever possible. Encourages resident to assist if possible.		
4.	Provides for resident's privacy with a curtain, screen, or door.		
5.	Puts on gloves.		
6.	Places paper towel on floor under drainage bag. Places graduate on paper towel.		
7.	Opens drain or clamp on bag. Allows urine to flow out of bag into graduate. Does not let clamp touch graduate.		
8.	When urine has drained, closes clamp. Using alcohol wipe, cleans drain clamp. Replaces drain in its holder on bag.		
9.	Notes amount and appearance of urine. Goes into bathroom. Places graduate on a flat surface and measures at eye level. Empties urine into toilet.		
10.	Cleans and stores measuring container. Discards paper towel.		

11.	Removes and disposes of gloves properly.		
12.	Leaves call light within resident's reach.		
13.	Washes hands.		
14.	Is courteous and respectful at all times.		
15.	Reports any changes in resident to nurse. Documents procedure and amount of urine (output) using facility guidelines.		

_____   _____
Date Reviewed   Instructor Signature

_____   _____
Date Performed   Instructor Signature

Applying a condom catheter

		yes	no
1.	Identifies self by name. Identifies resident and greets resident by name.		
2.	Washes hands.		
3.	Explains procedure to resident. Speaks clearly, slowly, and directly. Maintains face-to-face contact whenever possible. Encourages resident to assist if possible.		
4.	Provides for resident's privacy with a curtain, screen, or door.		
5.	Practices good body mechanics. Adjusts bed to safe working level. Locks bed wheels.		
6.	Lowers side rail on near side.		
7.	Lowers head of bed. Positions resident lying flat on back.		
8.	Removes or folds back top bedding. Keeps resident covered with bath blanket.		
9.	Puts on gloves.		
10.	Adjusts bath blanket to expose only genital area.		

Name: _____

11.	If condom catheter is present, gently removes it. Carefully disconnects condom from tube and immediately caps tube. Does not allow tube to touch anything. Places condom and tape in plastic bag.		
12.	Helps as necessary with perineal care.		
13.	Attaches collection bag to leg. Makes sure drain stays closed.		
14.	Moves pubic hair away from penis so it does not get rolled into condom.		
15.	Holds penis firmly. Places condom at tip of penis. Rolls towards base of penis. Leaves at least one inch of space between drainage tip and glans of penis. If resident is not circumcised, ensures that foreskin is in normal position.		
16.	Gently secures condom to penis with special tape provided or use self-adhesive. Applies in a spiral. Never wraps tape all the way around penis.		
17.	Connects catheter tip to drainage tubing. Does not touch tip to any object but drainage tubing. Makes sure tubing is not twisted or kinked.		
18.	Replaces top covers. Removes bath blanket. Makes resident comfortable.		
19.	Returns bed to low position. Ensures resident's safety. Returns side rails to ordered position. Removes privacy measures.		
20.	Disposes of plastic bag properly.		
21.	Removes and disposes of gloves properly.		
22.	Leaves call light within resident's reach.		
23.	Washes hands.		

24.	Is courteous and respectful at all times.		
25.	Reports any changes to nurse and documents procedure using facility guidelines.		

_____   _____
Date Reviewed   Instructor Signature

_____   _____
Date Performed   Instructor Signature

Collecting a routine urine specimen

		yes	no
1.	Identifies self by name. Identifies resident and greets resident by name.		
2.	Washes hands.		
3.	Explains procedure to resident. Speaks clearly, slowly, and directly. Maintains face-to-face contact whenever possible. Encourages resident to assist if possible.		
4.	Provides for resident's privacy with a curtain, screen, or door.		
5.	Puts on gloves.		
6.	Lowers side rail on near side.		
7.	Helps resident to bathroom or commode, or offers bedpan or urinal.		
8.	Has resident void into "hat," urinal, or bedpan. Asks resident not to put toilet paper or stool in with sample. Provides a plastic bag to discard toilet paper.		
9.	After urination, helps as necessary with perineal care. Helps resident wash his or her hands.		
10.	Removes and disposes of gloves properly. Washes hands.		
11.	Replaces bed covers. Makes resident comfortable.		
12.	Returns bed to low position. Ensures resident's safety. Returns side rails to ordered position. Removes privacy measures.		

		yes	no
13.	Puts on clean gloves.		
14.	Takes bedpan, urinal, or commode pail to bathroom.		
15.	Pours urine into specimen container until at least half full.		
16.	Covers urine container with its lid without touching inside of container. Wipes off outside with a paper towel, applies label, and bags specimen.		
17.	Discards extra urine and rinses and cleans equipment. Uses approved disinfectant if facility policy. Stores equipment.		
18.	Removes and disposes of gloves properly.		
19.	Leaves call light within resident's reach.		
20.	Washes hands.		
21.	Is courteous and respectful at all times.		
22.	Reports any changes to nurse and documents procedure using facility guidelines. Takes specimen and lab slip to designated place promptly.		

_____   _____
Date Reviewed   Instructor Signature

_____   _____
Date Performed   Instructor Signature

Collecting a clean-catch (midstream) urine specimen

		yes	no
1.	Identifies self by name. Identifies resident and greets resident by name.		
2.	Washes hands.		
3.	Explains procedure to resident. Speaks clearly, slowly, and directly. Maintains face-to-face contact whenever possible. Encourages resident to assist if possible.		
4.	Provides for resident's privacy with a curtain, screen, or door.		
5.	Lowers side rail on near side.		
6.	Puts on gloves.		
7.	Opens specimen kit without touching inside of container or lid.		
8.	If resident cannot clean his or her perineal area, does so. Uses towelettes or gauze and cleansing solution to clean area around meatus.		
	For females, separates labia. Wipes from front to back along one side. Discards towelette/gauze. With a new towelette or gauze, wipes from front to back along other side. Using a new towelette or gauze, wipes down middle.		
	For males, cleans head of penis. Uses circular motions with towelettes or gauze. Cleans thoroughly. Changes towelettes/gauze after each circular motion and discards after use. If man is uncircumcised, pulls back foreskin of penis before cleaning. Holds it back during urination. Makes sure it is pulled back down after collecting specimen.		
9.	Asks resident to urinate into bedpan, urinal, or toilet, and to stop before urination is complete.		
10.	Places container under urine stream. Does not touch resident's body with container. Has resident start urinating again. Fills container at least half full. Has resident stop urinating and removes container if possible. Has resident finish urinating in bedpan, urinal, or toilet.		
11.	After urination, helps as necessary with perineal care. Helps resident wash his or her hands.		
12.	Removes and disposes of gloves properly. Washes hands.		

Name: _____

13.	Replaces bed covers. Makes resident comfortable.		
14.	Returns bed to low position. Ensures resident's safety. Returns side rails to ordered position. Removes privacy measures.		
15.	Covers urine container with its lid without touching inside of container. Wipes off outside with a paper towel, applies label, and bags specimen.		
16.	If using a bedpan or urinal, discards extra urine. Rinses and cleans equipment. Uses approved disinfectant if facility policy. Stores equipment.		
17.	Removes and disposes of gloves properly.		
18.	Leaves call light within resident's reach.		
19.	Washes hands.		
20.	Is courteous and respectful at all times.		
21.	Reports any changes to nurse and documents procedure using facility guidelines. Takes specimen and lab slip to designated place promptly.		

_____   _____
Date Reviewed   Instructor Signature

_____   _____
Date Performed   Instructor Signature

Collecting a 24-hour urine specimen

		yes	no
1.	Identifies self by name. Identifies resident and greets resident by name.		
2.	Washes hands.		
3.	Explains procedure to resident. Speaks clearly, slowly, and directly. Maintains face-to-face contact whenever possible. Encourages resident to assist if possible.		

4.	Provides for resident's privacy with a curtain, screen, or door.		
5.	Places a sign on resident's bed to let all care team members know that a 24-hour specimen is being collected.		
6.	When starting collection, has resident completely empty bladder. Discards urine. Notes exact time of this voiding.		
7.	Puts on gloves each time resident voids. Measures I&O each time if needed.		
8.	Pours urine from bedpan, urinal, or toilet attachment into container. Stores specimen container according to facility policy.		

_____   _____
Date Reviewed   Instructor Signature

_____   _____
Date Performed   Instructor Signature

Testing urine with reagent strips

		yes	no
1.	Washes hands.		
2.	Puts on gloves.		
3.	Places paper towel on surface before setting urine specimen down.		
4.	Takes strip from the bottle and recaps bottle. Dips strip into specimen.		
5.	Follows manufacturer's instructions for when to remove strip. Removes strip at correct time.		
6.	Follows manufacturer's instructions for how long to wait after removing strip. After proper time has passed, compares strip with color chart on bottle. Does not touch bottle with strip.		
7.	Reads results.		
8.	Discards used items. Discards specimen in toilet.		
9.	Removes gloves.		

Name: _____

		yes	no
10.	Washes hands.		
11.	Records and reports results. Documents procedure using facility guidelines.		

_____   _____
Date Reviewed   Instructor Signature

_____   _____
Date Performed   Instructor Signature

Giving a vaginal douche

		yes	no
1.	Identifies self by name. Identifies resident and greets resident by name.		
2.	Washes hands.		
3.	Explains procedure to resident. Speaks clearly, slowly, and directly. Maintains face-to-face contact whenever possible. Encourages resident to assist if possible.		
4.	Provides for resident's privacy with a curtain, screen, or door.		
5.	Practices good body mechanics. Adjusts bed to safe working level. Locks bed wheels.		
6.	Lowers side rail on near side.		
7.	Lowers head of bed. Positions resident lying flat on back.		
8.	Applies gloves.		
9.	Covers resident with a bath blanket. Asks her to hold it while pulling down top covers underneath. Does not expose more of resident than necessary.		
10.	Places a bed protector under resident's buttocks and hips.		
11.	Hangs prepared vaginal irrigation bag on IV pole and lowers pole so that bag is 12 inches above resident's perineal area.		
12.	Removes resident's pants or pajama bottoms, exposing only as much of resident's body as necessary.		
13.	Places bedpan under resident and makes sure she is in dorsal recumbent position.		
14.	Opens clamp and allows a little water to run from tubing into bedpan.		
15.	Lubricates tip of tubing.		
16.	Inserts nozzle slowly and gently into vagina about two to three inches.		
17.	Begins slow flow of water or fluid by releasing clamp. Before vaginal irrigation bag is empty, clamps tubing.		
18.	Removes tubing slowly and gently and places tubing tip inside top of bag.		
19.	Raises head of bed so that resident is in a semi-sitting position on bedpan.		
20.	Removes bedpan and covers it. Removes bed protector.		
21.	Dries perineal area and buttocks and replaces clothing or gown. Removes bath blanket and replaces top covers.		
22.	Returns bed to low position. Ensures resident's safety. Returns side rails to ordered position. Removes privacy measures.		
23.	Makes resident comfortable.		
24.	Brings bedpan to bathroom and checks contents for anything unusual. Empties bedpan.		
25.	Rinses bedpan and pours rinse water into toilet. Uses approved disinfectant if facility policy. Returns to proper storage.		
26.	Places soiled linens, clothing and bed protector in proper containers.		
27.	Removes and disposes of gloves properly.		
28.	Leaves call light within resident's reach.		

29.	Washes hands.		
30.	Is courteous and respectful at all times.		
31.	Reports any changes to nurse and documents procedure using facility guidelines.		

_____ _____
Date Reviewed   Instructor Signature

_____ _____
Date Performed   Instructor Signature

Applying warm moist compresses

		yes	no
1.	Identifies self by name. Identifies resident and greets resident by name.		
2.	Washes hands.		
3.	Explains procedure to resident. Speaks clearly, slowly, and directly. Maintains face-to-face contact whenever possible. Encourages resident to assist if possible.		
4.	Provides for resident's privacy with a curtain, screen, or door.		
5.	Fills basin one-half to two-thirds full with warm water. Tests water temperature with thermometer or wrist. Ensures it is safe. Has resident check water temperature. Adjusts if necessary.		
6.	Soaks washcloth in water. Wrings it out. Immediately applies it to area needing a warm compress. Notes time. Quickly covers washcloth with plastic wrap and towel.		
7.	Checks area every five minutes. Removes compress if area is red or numb or if resident has pain or discomfort. Changes compress if cooling occurs. Removes compress after 20 minutes.		

8.	If using commercial warm compress, follows package directions and nurse's instructions.		
9.	Removes privacy measures. Makes resident comfortable.		
10.	Empties, rinses, and wipes basin. Returns to proper storage. Discards plastic wrap.		
11.	Places soiled clothing and linens in appropriate containers.		
12.	Leaves call light within resident's reach.		
13.	Washes hands.		
14.	Is courteous and respectful at all times.		
15.	Reports any changes to nurse and documents procedure using facility guidelines.		

_____ _____
Date Reviewed   Instructor Signature

_____ _____
Date Performed   Instructor Signature

Administering warm soaks

		yes	no
1.	Identifies self by name. Identifies resident and greets resident by name.		
2.	Washes hands.		
3.	Explains procedure to resident. Speaks clearly, slowly, and directly. Maintains face-to-face contact whenever possible. Encourages resident to assist if possible.		
4.	Provides for resident's privacy with a curtain, screen, or door.		
5.	Fills basin half full of warm water. Tests water temperature with thermometer or wrist, and ensures it is safe. Has resident check water temperature. Adjusts if necessary.		

6.	Immerses body part in basin. Pads edge of basin with a towel if needed. Uses a bath blanket to cover resident if needed for extra warmth.		
7.	Checks water temperature every five minutes. Adds warm water as needed to maintain temperature. Never adds water warmer than 105°F. Tells resident not to add warm water. Observes area for redness. Discontinue soak if resident has pain or discomfort.		
8.	Soaks for 15-20 minutes, or as ordered.		
9.	Removes basin. Uses towel to dry resident.		
10.	Removes privacy measures. Makes resident comfortable.		
11.	Empties, rinses, and wipes basin. Returns to proper storage.		
12.	Places soiled clothing and linens in appropriate containers.		
13.	Leaves call light within resident's reach.		
14.	Washes hands.		
15.	Is courteous and respectful at all times.		
16.	Reports any changes to nurse and documents procedure using facility guidelines.		

_____ _____
Date Reviewed   Instructor Signature

_____ _____
Date Performed   Instructor Signature

Applying an Aquamatic K-Pad®

		yes	no
1.	Identifies self by name. Identifies resident and greets resident by name.		
2.	Washes hands.		

3.	Explains procedure to resident. Speaks clearly, slowly, and directly. Maintains face-to-face contact whenever possible. Encourages resident to assist if possible.		
4.	Provides for resident's privacy with a curtain, screen, or door.		
5.	Makes sure surface on bedside table is dry and places control unit on bedside table. Makes sure cords are not frayed or damaged and that tubing between pad and unit is intact.		
6.	Removes cover of control unit to check level of water. If it is low, fills it with distilled water to fill line.		
7.	Puts cover of control unit back in place.		
8.	Plugs unit in and turns unit on. If temperature was not pre-set, checks with nurse for proper temperature. If setting temperature, removes key after doing so. Places key in proper place.		
9.	Places pad in cover. Does not pin pad to cover.		
10.	Uncovers area to be treated. Places covered pad. Notes time. Makes sure tubing is not hanging below bed and is not kinked.		
11.	Returns to check area every five minutes. Removes pad if area is red or numb or if resident reports pain or discomfort.		
12.	Checks water level. Refills with distilled water to fill line when necessary.		
13.	Turns off unit and removes pad after 20 minutes.		
14.	Removes privacy measures. Makes resident comfortable.		
15.	Returns K-Pad® to proper storage.		
16.	Places used linen in appropriate container.		

17.	Leaves call light within resident's reach.		
18.	Washes hands.		
19.	Is courteous and respectful at all times.		
20.	Reports any changes to nurse and documents procedure using facility guidelines.		

Date Reviewed _____ Instructor Signature _____

Date Performed _____ Instructor Signature _____

Assisting with a sitz bath

		yes	no
1.	Identifies self by name. Identifies resident and greets resident by name.		
2.	Washes hands.		
3.	Explains procedure to resident. Speaks clearly, slowly, and directly. Maintains face-to-face contact whenever possible. Encourages resident to assist if possible.		
4.	Provides for resident's privacy with a curtain, screen, or door.		
5.	Puts on gloves.		
6.	Fills sitz bath two-thirds full with warm water. Places disposable sitz bath on toilet seat. Follows care plan. Checks water temperature using bath thermometer.		
7.	Helps resident undress and get seated on sitz bath. Uses valve on tubing connected to bag to fill sitz bath again with warm water when needed.		
8.	Stays with resident if needed. If leaving room, checks on resident every five minutes. Makes sure resident knows how to use emergency pull cord in bathroom if needed.		

9.	Helps resident out of sitz bath in 20 minutes. Provides towels. Helps with dressing if needed.		
10.	Empties, rinses, and wipes sitz bath container. Returns to proper storage.		
11.	Places soiled clothing and linens in appropriate containers.		
12.	Removes privacy measures. Makes resident comfortable.		
13.	Removes and disposes of gloves properly.		
14.	Leaves call light within resident's reach.		
15.	Washes hands.		
16.	Is courteous and respectful at all times.		
17.	Reports any changes to nurse and documents procedure using facility guidelines.		

Date Reviewed _____ Instructor Signature _____

Date Performed _____ Instructor Signature _____

Applying ice packs

		yes	no
1.	Identifies self by name. Identifies resident and greets resident by name.		
2.	Washes hands.		
3.	Explains procedure to resident. Speaks clearly, slowly, and directly. Maintains face-to-face contact whenever possible. Encourages resident to assist if possible.		
4.	Provides for resident's privacy with a curtain, screen, or door.		
5.	Practices good body mechanics. Locks bed wheels.		
6.	Fills plastic bag or ice pack one-half to two-thirds full with crushed ice and seals. Removes excess air. Covers bag or ice pack with towel or cover.		

7.	Applies bag to area as ordered. Notes time. Uses another towel to cover bag if it is too cold.		
8.	Checks area after five minutes for blisters or pale, white, or gray skin. Stops treatment if resident reports numbness or pain.		
9.	Removes ice and water after 20 minutes or as ordered.		
10.	Removes privacy measures. Makes resident comfortable.		
11.	Empties and stores ice pack.		
12.	Places used linen in appropriate container.		
13.	Leaves call light within resident's reach.		
14.	Washes hands.		
15.	Is courteous and respectful at all times.		
16.	Reports any changes to nurse and documents procedure using facility guidelines.		

_____ _____
Date Reviewed   Instructor Signature

_____ _____
Date Performed   Instructor Signature

Assisting the nurse with changing a non-sterile dressing

		yes	no
1.	Identifies self by name. Identifies resident and greets resident by name.		
2.	Washes hands.		
3.	Explains procedure to resident. Speaks clearly, slowly, and directly. Maintains face-to-face contact whenever possible. Encourages resident to assist if possible.		
4.	Provides for resident's privacy with a curtain, screen, or door.		
5.	Keeps plastic bag close by for immediate disposal of old dressing materials.		

6.	Opens packages for nurse or cuts strips of tape if asked. Cuts pieces of tape long enough to secure dressing. Opens gauze square packages without touching inside of gauze. If asked to set package down, places opened package on a clean, flat surface.		
7.	Puts on gloves.		
8.	Only exposes area where dressing will be changed. Disposes of used dressing in proper container.		
9.	Removes and disposes of gloves in plastic bag.		
10.	Washes hands.		
11.	Puts on new gloves. Assists nurse with application of new dressing as directed.		
12.	Removes privacy measures.		
13.	Removes and disposes of gloves properly.		
14.	Leaves call light within resident's reach.		
15.	Washes hands.		
16.	Is courteous and respectful at all times.		
17.	Reports any changes to nurse and documents procedure using facility guidelines.		

_____ _____
Date Reviewed   Instructor Signature

_____ _____
Date Performed   Instructor Signature

Applying sterile gloves

		yes	no
1.	Washes hands.		
2.	Removes outer wrapper from gloves. Places inner wrapper on clean surface with word "Left" on left side and word "Right" on right side.		

Name: _____

3.	Slowly opens inner wrapper, only touching small flaps of wrapper.		
4.	Picks up first glove by bottom end of cuff.		
5.	Slips fingers into glove without touching outside of glove. Waits to adjust glove until second glove is on other hand.		
6.	Slips gloved hand into second glove in area under cuff.		
7.	Slowly slips fingers of ungloved hand into second glove, and pulls it completely over hand and wrist.		
8.	With gloved second hand, finishes pulling first glove up and over wrist. Adjusts fingers if any adjustment is necessary.		
9.	If either glove has a tear in it, stops and starts again with second set of sterile gloves.		
10.	Keeps gloved hands in front of self and above level of waist at all times.		
11.	Assists nurse with sterile procedure.		

_____ _____
Date Reviewed   Instructor Signature

_____ _____
Date Performed   Instructor Signature

Putting knee-high elastic stockings on a resident

		yes	no
1.	Identifies self by name. Identifies resident and greets resident by name.		
2.	Washes hands.		
3.	Explains procedure to resident. Speaks clearly, slowly, and directly. Maintains face-to-face contact whenever possible. Encourages resident to assist if possible.		

4.	Provides for resident's privacy with a curtain, screen, or door.		
5.	Practices good body mechanics. Adjusts bed to safe working level. Locks bed wheels.		
6.	Lowers side rail on near side.		
7.	Exposes no more than one leg at a time. Takes one stocking and turns it inside-out at least to heel area.		
8.	Gently places foot of stocking over toes, foot, and heel.		
9.	Gently pulls top of stocking over foot, heel, and leg.		
10.	Makes sure there are no twists or wrinkles in stocking after it is on leg and that opening in stocking that allows observation of skin color is either on top or bottom of toe area, depending upon manufacturer. Checks toes for possible pressure from stocking and adjusts as needed.		
11.	Repeats steps 6 through 10 for other leg.		
12.	Makes resident comfortable.		
13.	Returns bed to low position. Ensures resident's safety. Returns side rails to ordered position. Removes privacy measures.		
14.	Leaves call light within resident's reach.		
15.	Washes hands.		
16.	Is courteous and respectful at all times.		
17.	Reports any changes to nurse and documents procedure using facility guidelines.		

_____ _____
Date Reviewed   Instructor Signature

_____ _____
Date Performed   Instructor Signature

Name: _____

Collecting a sputum specimen

		yes	no
1.	Identifies self by name. Identifies resident and greets resident by name.		
2.	Washes hands.		
3.	Explains procedure to resident. Speaks clearly, slowly, and directly. Maintains face-to-face contact whenever possible. Encourages resident to assist if possible.		
4.	Provides for resident's privacy with a curtain, screen, or door.		
5.	Puts on mask and gloves. If resident has known or suspected TB or another infectious disease, wears proper mask when collecting a sputum specimen.		
6.	Asks resident to rinse mouth with water. Assists as necessary. Has resident spit rinse water in emesis basin or sink.		
7.	Asks resident to cough deeply, so that sputum comes up from lungs. Gives resident tissues to cover mouth. Asks resident to spit sputum into container.		
8.	Covers container tightly when about two tablespoons of sputum have been obtained. Wipes any sputum off outside of container with tissues. Discards tissues. Applies label and bags specimen.		
9.	Removes and disposes of gloves and mask properly.		
10.	Leaves call light within resident's reach.		
11.	Washes hands.		
12.	Is courteous and respectful at all times.		
13.	Reports any changes to nurse and documents procedure using facility guidelines. Takes specimen container and lab slip to designated place promptly.		

Date Reviewed _____ Instructor Signature _____

Date Performed _____ Instructor Signature _____

Applying elastic bandages

		yes	no
1.	Identifies self by name. Identifies resident and greets resident by name.		
2.	Washes hands.		
3.	Explains procedure to resident. Speaks clearly, slowly, and directly. Maintains face-to-face contact whenever possible. Encourages resident to assist if possible.		
4.	Provides for resident's privacy with a curtain, screen, or door.		
5.	Practices good body mechanics. Adjusts bed to safe working level. Locks bed wheels.		
6.	Lowers side rail on near side.		
7.	Avoids trauma or pain to resident throughout procedure.		
8.	Assists resident to get into supine (flat on back) position.		
9.	Exposes only part to be bandaged.		
10.	Holds rolled bandage with one hand and with other hand puts loose end on top of extremity.		
11.	Wraps extremity beginning at spot furthest from heart to allow extra fluid to flow to heart and leave area. For wrist, begins wrapping at hand; for ankle, begins at foot.		

12.	Wraps bandage once around beginning spot and turns over tip so that an anchor is made.		
13.	Wraps one more time around spot where anchor lies and begins slowly wrapping in over-lapping spirals up extremity.		
14.	Smoothes out entire bandage, removing any wrinkles.		
15.	Secures bandage with self-clo-sure, clip, safety pin, or tape.		
16.	Straightens all linens.		
17.	Removes and re-applies ban-dage as directed. Washes and dries bandages as necessary.		
18.	Makes resident comfortable.		
19.	Returns bed to low position. Ensures resident's safety. Returns side rails to ordered position. Removes privacy measures.		
20.	Leaves call light within resi-dent's reach.		
21.	Washes hands.		
22.	Is courteous and respectful at all times.		
23.	Reports any changes to nurse and documents procedure using facility guidelines.		

_____ _____
Date Reviewed   Instructor Signature

_____ _____
Date Performed   Instructor Signature

Caring for eyeglasses

		yes	no
1.	Identifies self by name. Identifies resident and greets resident by name.		
2.	Washes hands.		

3.	Explains procedure to resident. Speaks clearly, slowly, and directly. Maintains face-to-face contact whenever possible. Encourages resident to assist if possible.		
4.	Provides for resident's privacy with a curtain, screen, or door.		
5.	Gently removes eyeglasses and places in emesis basin.		
6.	Lines sink with towel.		
7.	Cleans eyeglasses over lined sink. Washes glass lenses in lukewarm water and rinses. Cleans plastic lenses with cleaning fluid and a lens cloth. Observes for loose screws or loose or broken lenses.		
8.	Dries with soft, 100% cotton cloth or special lens cloth.		
9.	Gently assists resident to replace eyeglasses on face. Places over ears and positions comfortably. Observes for prop-er fit.		
10.	Removes privacy measures. Makes resident comfortable.		
11.	Leaves call light within resi-dent's reach.		
12.	Washes hands.		
13.	Is courteous and respectful at all times.		
14.	Reports any changes to nurse and documents procedure using facility guidelines.		

_____ _____
Date Reviewed   Instructor Signature

_____ _____
Date Performed   Instructor Signature

Providing foot care

		yes	no
	Supports foot and ankle throughout procedure.		

Name: _____

1.	Identifies self by name. Identifies resident and greets resident by name.		
2.	Washes hands.		
3.	Explains procedure to resident. Speaks clearly, slowly, and directly. Maintains face-to-face contact whenever possible. Encourages resident to assist if possible.		
4.	Provides for resident's privacy with a curtain, screen, or door.		
5.	Practices good body mechanics. If resident is in bed, locks bed wheels.		
6.	Fills basin halfway with warm water. Tests water temperature with thermometer or wrist. Ensures it is safe. Has resident check water temperature. Adjusts if necessary.		
7.	Places basin on bath mat.		
8.	Removes resident's socks. Completely submerges resident's feet in water. Soaks feet for five to ten minutes.		
9.	Puts on gloves.		
10.	Removes one foot from water. Washes entire foot with soapy washcloth.		
11.	Rinses entire foot, including between toes.		
12.	Dries entire foot, including between toes.		
13.	Repeats steps 10 through 12 for other foot.		
14.	Puts lotion in hand. Warms lotion by rubbing hands together.		
15.	Massages lotion into feet (top and bottom), except between toes, removing excess with a towel.		
16.	Assists resident to replace socks.		
17.	Makes resident comfortable.		

18.	Returns bed to low position. Ensures resident's safety. Removes privacy measures.		
19.	Empties, rinses, and wipes basin. Returns to proper storage.		
20.	Disposes of soiled linen in proper container.		
21.	Removes and disposes of gloves properly.		
22.	Leaves call light within resident's reach.		
23.	Washes hands.		
24.	Is courteous and respectful at all times.		
25.	Reports any changes to nurse and documents procedure using facility guidelines.		

_____ _____
Date Reviewed   Instructor Signature

_____ _____
Date Performed   Instructor Signature

Assisting with ambulation for resident with cane, walker or crutches

		yes	no
1.	Identifies self by name. Identifies resident and greets resident by name.		
2.	Washes hands.		
3.	Explains procedure to resident. Speaks clearly, slowly, and directly. Maintains face-to-face contact whenever possible. Encourages resident to assist if possible.		
4.	Provides for resident's privacy with a curtain, screen, or door.		
5.	Before ambulating, puts on and properly fastens non-skid footwear on resident.		
6.	Adjusts bed to a low position so that resident's feet are flat on floor. Locks bed wheels.		

Name: _____

7.	Stands in front of and faces resident.		
8.	Braces resident's lower extremities. Bends knees. If resident has a weak knee, braces resident's knee against NA's knee.		
9.	Places transfer belt around resident's waist and grasps belt, while helping resident to stand.		
10.	Helps as needed with ambulation.		
11.	Walks slightly behind and on weaker side of resident. Holds transfer belt if used.		
12.	Watches for obstacles in path. Asks resident to look ahead, not down at his feet.		
13.	Encourages resident to rest if tired. Lets resident set pace. Discusses how far he plans to go based on care plan.		
14.	Removes transfer belt. Helps resident to a position of comfort and safety in bed or chair.		
15.	If in bed, returns bed to low position. Ensures resident's safety. Removes privacy measures.		
16.	Leaves call light within resident's reach.		
17.	Washes hands.		
18.	Is courteous and respectful at all times.		
19.	Reports any changes to nurse and documents procedure using facility guidelines.		

_____   _____
Date Reviewed   Instructor Signature

_____   _____
Date Performed   Instructor Signature

Assisting with passive range of motion exercises

		yes	no
1.	Identifies self by name. Identifies resident and greets resident by name.		
2.	Washes hands.		
3.	Explains procedure to resident. Speaks clearly, slowly, and directly. Maintains face-to-face contact whenever possible. Encourages resident to assist if possible.		
4.	Provides for resident's privacy with a curtain, screen, or door.		
5.	Practices good body mechanics. Adjusts bed to a safe level. Locks bed wheels.		
6.	Lowers side rail on near side.		
7.	Positions resident lying supine on bed. Positions body in good alignment.		
8.	Repeats each exercise at least 3 times.		
9.	**Shoulder**. Supports resident's arm at elbow and wrist while performing ROM for shoulder. Places one hand under elbow and other hand under wrist. Raises straightened arm from side position forward to above head and returns arm to side of body. Raises arm to side position above head and returns arm to side of body.		
10.	**Elbow**. Holds wrist with one hand. Holds elbow with other hand. Bends elbow so that hand touches shoulder on same side. Straightens arm. Exercises forearm by moving it so palm is facing downward and then upward.		

11.	**Wrist**. Holds wrist with one hand. Uses fingers of other hand to help joint through motions. Bends hand down. Bends hand backwards. Turns hand in direction of thumb. Then turns hand in direction of little finger.		
12.	**Thumb**. Moves thumb away from index finger. Moves thumb back next to index finger. Touches each fingertip with thumb. Bends thumb into palm and out to side.		
13.	**Fingers**. Makes hand into a fist. Gently straightens out fist. Spreads fingers and thumb far apart from each other. Brings fingers back next to each other.		
14.	**Hip**. Supports leg by placing one hand under knee and one under ankle. Straightens leg. Raises it gently upward. Moves leg away from other leg. Moves leg toward other leg. Gently turns leg inward. Turns leg outward.		
15.	**Knees**. Supports resident's leg under knee and ankle. Bends knee to point of resistance. Returns leg to normal position.		
16.	**Ankles**. Supports foot and ankle close to bed. Pushes/pulls foot up toward head. Pushes/pulls foot down, with toes pointed down. Turns inside of foot inward toward body. Bends sole of foot away from body.		
17.	**Toes**. Curls and straightens toes. Gently spreads toes apart.		
18.	While supporting limbs, moves all joints gently, slowly, and smoothly through range of motion to point of resistance. Stops exercises if any pain occurs.		

19.	Returns bed to low position. Ensures resident's safety. Returns side rails to ordered position. Removes privacy measures.		
20.	Leaves call light within resident's reach.		
21.	Washes hands.		
22.	Is courteous and respectful at all times.		
23.	Reports any changes to nurse and documents procedure using facility guidelines.		

_____   _____
Date Reviewed   Instructor Signature

_____   _____
Date Performed   Instructor Signature

Postmortem care

		yes	no
1.	Identifies resident.		
2.	Washes hands.		
3.	Explains procedure to resident's family and asks them to step outside. Is courteous, respectful, and compassionate at all times.		
4.	Provides for privacy with a curtain, screen, or door.		
5.	Practices good body mechanics. Adjusts bed to safe working level. Locks bed wheels.		
6.	Avoids trauma to resident's body throughout procedure. Treats body with utmost respect.		
7.	Applies gloves.		
8.	Turns off any oxygen, suction, or other equipment, if directed by nurse. Does not remove any tubes or other equipment.		
9.	Gently closes eyes without pressure.		
10.	Positions body in good alignment, on back with legs straight. Folds arms across abdomen.		

11.	Closes mouth. Places rolled towel under chin.		
12.	Gently bathes body, being careful to avoid bruising. Replaces any dressings only if directed to do so.		
13.	Combs or brushes hair gently without tugging.		
14.	Places drainage pads where needed.		
15.	Puts a clean gown on body.		
16.	Covers body to just over shoulders with sheet. Does not cover face or head.		
17.	Tidies room so family may visit.		
18.	Removes all used supplies and linen.		
19.	Follows facility's policy for handling or removing personal items. Has a witness if personal items are removed or given to a family member.		
20.	Removes gloves and washes hands.		
21.	Turns lights down and allows family to enter and spend private time with resident. Returns bed to low position.		
22.	Returns after family departs and applies clean gloves.		
23.	Places shroud on resident and follows instructions on completing ID tags.		
24.	Removes gloves and washes hands.		
25.	Reports any changes to nurse and documents procedure using facility guidelines.		

_____   _____
Date Reviewed   Instructor Signature

_____   _____
Date Performed   Instructor Signature

Practice Exam

1. One task commonly assigned to nursing assistants is:
   a. Inserting and removing tubes
   b. Changing sterile dressings
   c. Helping residents with toileting needs
   d. Giving tube feedings

2. The most important member of the care team is:
   a. The nursing assistant
   b. The nurse
   c. The physician
   d. The resident

3. All of the following are examples of ethical behavior for a nursing assistant EXCEPT:
   a. Graciously accepting gifts and tips from residents and their families and friends
   b. Keeping resident and staff information confidential
   c. Documenting care given accurately and promptly
   d. Treating residents with respect and empathy

4. If a nursing assistant suspects that a resident is being abused, he should:
   a. Report it to his supervisor immediately..
   b. Confront the abuser.
   c. Keep watching until he is sure abuse is occurring.
   d. Ask the resident's friends if the resident is being abused.

5. A nursing assistant may share confidential resident information with:
   a. The resident's friends and family
   b. Other members of the care team
   c. Anyone who asks
   d. Other residents

6. Which of the following is an objective statement?
   a. Mr. Harris has a rash on his back.
   b. Mrs. Carpenter has been having headaches lately.
   c. Mr. Jansson says his medication makes him nauseous.
   d. Ms. Peters' knees hurt when she is walking.

7. When may a nursing assistant hit a resident?
   a. When the resident becomes combative
   b. When the resident threatens to hit the nursing assistant or someone else
   c. Only if the resident hits the nursing assistant first
   d. Never

8. All of the following are methods of communicating with a resident with an impairment EXCEPT:
   a. Use the face of an imaginary clock to explain position of objects to a visually impaired resident
   b. Exaggerate pronunciation of words when speaking to a resident with hearing impairment
   c. Speak slowly and calmly to a resident who is fearful or anxious
   d. Encourage social interaction for residents who are depressed

9. Psychosocial needs include:
   a. Need for activity
   b. Need for sleep and rest
   c. Need for love and acceptance
   d. Need for clothing and shelter

Name: _____

10. If a nursing assistant encounters a sexual situation between two consenting residents, he should:
    a. Provide privacy
    b. Ask the residents to stop
    c. Tell his supervisor
    d. Tell other residents

11. All of the following are reasons that the elderly are at a higher risk for infection EXCEPT:
    a. The immune system becomes stronger with age.
    b. Elderly people are hospitalized more often.
    c. Recovery from illness takes longer for older people.
    d. Thinner skin and limited mobility increase the risk of pressure sores.

12. The single most important thing a nursing assistant can do to prevent the spread of disease is to:
    a. Keep fingernails short and clean.
    b. Wash hands.
    c. Apply and use PPE correctly.
    d. Practice Standard Precautions on every resident.

13. Most of the accidents in a facility are related to:
    a. Burns and scalds
    b. Failing to identify residents before performing care or serving food
    c. Choking
    d. Falls

14. All of the following are complications of restraint use EXCEPT:
    a. Increased blood circulation
    b. Pressure sores
    c. Muscle atrophy
    d. Increased agitation

15. Symptoms of myocardial infarction that are experienced more often by women include:
    a. Back or jaw pain
    b. Dizziness
    c. Cold and clammy skin
    d. Anxiety and a sense of doom

16. Symptoms that a stroke is beginning include all of the following EXCEPT:
    a. Blurred vision
    b. Ringing in the ears
    c. Slurring of words
    d. Increased pulse rate

17. One way a nursing assistant can help a new resident adjust to life in a facility is:
    a. Tell the resident how much work it is to care for her.
    b. Hide any mistakes you make so that residents will feel more confident in your work.
    c. Listen to residents if they want to express their feelings.
    d. Push residents to join in activities even if they don't want to.

18. All of the following can improve a resident's ability to sleep EXCEPT:
    a. Keep doors open at night.
    b. Change soiled bed linens and clothing as soon as possible.
    c. Report to nurse if room temperature is a problem.
    d. Observe and report signs of pain promptly.

19. A bed made while the resident is in it is:
    a. An open bed
    b. A closed bed
    c. An occupied bed
    d. A surgical bed

20. All of the following are components of proper body mechanics EXCEPT:
    a. Use a wide but balanced stance to increase support.
    b. Lift with the back muscles to decrease stress on the legs.
    c. Face what you are lifting.
    d. Push or pull when possible rather than lifting.

21. All of the following are true about ambulation EXCEPT:
    a. An ambulatory resident can get out of bed and walk.
    b. Ambulation helps residents maintain independence.
    c. Ambulation can make it hard for a resident to sleep or relax.
    d. A person who is just starting to ambulate should only walk for short distances.

22. One way to promote residents' dignity during personal care is to:
    a. Decide how often and when a resident should be bathed.
    b. Choose residents' clothing and jewelry for them so they don't have to worry about it.
    c. If a resident is taking a long time performing a task, do it for him.
    d. Always provide privacy when giving personal care.

23. Observing for changes in residents' skin is especially important in the prevention of:
    a. Falls and other accidents
    b. Pressure sores
    c. Edema
    d. Weight loss

24. If a nursing assistant cannot obtain a reading when measuring vital signs, she should:
    a. Guess
    b. Use the previous reading for that resident
    c. Leave that space in the chart blank
    d. Tell the nurse

25. An oral temperature may be taken for a resident who:
    a. Is unconscious
    b. Is confused or disoriented
    c. Has an injury to an extremity
    d. Has facial trauma

26. According to the USDA's MyPyramid, which food group should make up the largest proportion of the diet?
    a. Grains
    b. Meat and beans
    c. Vegetables
    d. Milk products

27. All of the following are guidelines for making dining enjoyable for residents EXCEPT:
    a. Assist residents with grooming requests.
    b. Honor requests to seat residents by their friends.
    c. Position residents at a 45° angle for eating.
    d. Serve food promptly to maintain the correct temperature.

28. Normal changes of aging in the gastrointestinal system include:
    a. Increased ability to taste
    b. More frequent constipation
    c. Increased production of saliva and digestive fluids
    d. Presence of blood or mucus in stool

29. A build-up of dry, hardened feces in the rectum that results from unrelieved constipation is:
    a. Fecal impaction
    b. Incontinence
    c. Ulcer
    d. GERD

30. One way for a nursing assistant to promote normal urination is:
    a. Reduce residents' intake of fluids.
    b. Discourage activity and exercise.
    c. Provide plenty of privacy and time for elimination.
    d. Ask residents to wait as long as they can before going to the bathroom.

31. All of the following are guidelines for dealing with episodes of incontinence EXCEPT:
    a. Know residents' routines and urinary habits.
    b. Answer call lights promptly.
    c. Refer to incontinence briefs as "diapers."
    d. Provide privacy for episodes of incontinence.

32. All of the following may affect a resident's sexual activity EXCEPT:
    a. Sexual desire goes away as a person ages.
    b. Illness may reduce or affect the ability to perform sexually.
    c. Depression
    d. Lack of privacy

Name: _____

33. A burn in which some skin damage and blistering occurs but the muscle and bone are not affected is a:
a. First degree burn
b. Second degree burn
c. Third degree burn
d. Scald

34. Heat applications may have all of the following beneficial effects EXCEPT:
a. Relief of pain
b. Relief of muscular tension
c. Decreased blood flow due to constriction of vessels
d. Increased waste removal from area

35. What does a diagnosis of prehypertension mean?
a. The person has high blood pressure.
b. The person does not have high blood pressure now but is likely to in the future.
c. The person has low blood pressure.
d. The person does not have low blood pressure now but is likely to in the future.

36. When should anti-embolic stockings be applied?
a. In the morning
b. In the afternoon
c. Right before the resident goes to bed
d. During or after surgery

37. Residents with COPD might be fearful of:
a. Not being able to breathe
b. Not being able to walk
c. Not being able to eat
d. Not being able to remember friends and family members

38. A resident with tuberculosis must:
a. Take as little of prescribed medication as possible.
b. Take all of the prescribed medication.
c. Keep the doors to the airborne infection isolation room open.
d. Use an inhaler.

39. Osteoporosis can be caused by all of the following EXCEPT:
a. Brain damage
b. Lack of calcium in the diet
c. Loss of estrogen
d. Reduced mobility or lack of regular exercise

40. Strategies for better communication with residents with Alzheimer's disease include:
a. Touch the resident before speaking to him.
b. Reduce background noise.
c. Look away from the resident while talking to him.
d. Talk about several different subjects at the same time.

41. If a resident with AD has hallucinations, a nursing assistant should:
a. Ignore the hallucination and reassure the resident.
b. Pretend to see what the resident is seeing.
c. Tell the resident that she is imagining things.
d. Tell the resident's family.

42. Diabetes is more common in people who:
a. Have a family history of the illness
b. Are under the age of 50
c. Are unable to get out of bed
d. Are underweight

43. Care guidelines for diabetes include all of the following EXCEPT:
a. Observe skin carefully for sores, blisters or any other breaks in the skin.
b. Perform foot care carefully as directed.
c. Discourage diabetic residents from exercising.
d. Carefully follow diet instructions.

44. HIV/AIDS can be transmitted by:
a. Unprotected or poorly protected sexual contact with an infected person
b. Hugging an infected person
c. Drinking water from the same fountain as an infected person
d. Being bitten by a mosquito

45. A _____ tumor is non-cancerous; a _____ tumor is cancerous.
    a. Malignant, benign
    b. Benign, malignant
    c. Malignant, metastasized
    d. Metastasized, malignant

46. All of the following are negative effects of inactivity EXCEPT:
    a. Pressure sores and slow-healing wounds
    b. Blood clots
    c. Increased metabolism
    d. Depression or insomnia

47. Devices applied externally to a limb for support and protection are called:
    a. Assistive devices
    b. Adaptive devices
    c. Orthotic devices
    d. Trochanter rolls

48. Guidelines for caring for residents who are on a ventilator include:
    a. Do not speak to residents on a ventilator while providing care.
    b. Assume that the resident cannot understand what is going on around her.
    c. Enter the room often so the resident can see you.
    d. Residents on a ventilator will not need oral care.

49. Goals of hospice care include all of the following EXCEPT:
    a. Curing the resident's disease
    b. Using a holistic approach to care
    c. Focusing on soothing and comfort care
    d. Helping the family obtain financial counseling and legal assistance

50. Employee evaluations include all of the following EXCEPT:
    a. Evaluation of employee's knowledge, conflict resolution, and team effort
    b. Hostile criticism
    c. Constructive criticism
    d. Ideas for solving problems